A Practical Guide to Writing a Ruth L. Kirschstein NRSA Grant

T0296632

A Practical Guide to Writing a Ruth L. Kirschstein NRSA Grant

Second Edition

Andrew D. Hollenbach, Ph.D.

Professor, Department of Genetics
Louisiana State University Health Sciences Center
New Orleans, LA, United States

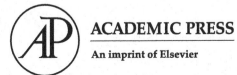

ACADEMIC PRESS

An imprint of Elsevier

Academic Press is an imprint of Elsevier
125 London Wall, London EC2Y 5AS, United Kingdom
525 B Street, Suite 1650, San Diego, CA 92101-4495, United States
50 Hampshire Street, 5th Floor, Cambridge, MA 02139, United States
The Boulevard, Langford Lane, Kidlington, Oxford OX5 1GB, United Kingdom

British Library Cataloguing-in-Publication Data
A catalogue record for this book is available from the British Library

Library of Congress Cataloging-in-Publication Data
A catalog record for this book is available from the Library of Congress

ISBN: 978-0-12-815336-9

For Information on all Academic Press publications
visit our website at https://www.elsevier.com/books-and-journals

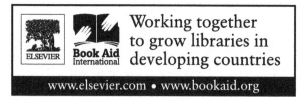

Working together
to grow libraries in
developing countries

www.elsevier.com • www.bookaid.org

Publisher: Mica Haley
Acquisition Editor: Mary Preap
Editorial Project Manager: Mary Preap
Production Project Manager: Punithavathy Govindaradjane
Designer: Christian J. Bilbow

Typeset by MPS Limited, Chennai, India

Cover image of Dr. Ruth Kirschstein courtesy of the NIH; Photo credit: Bill Branson

I would like to dedicate this book to my friend and colleague Erica Golemis, PhD, a woman who has been a true mentor to me throughout my scientific career. Her advice, guidance, support, and friendship have helped me to become the educator I am today.

CONTENTS

It has been nearly 5 years since I completed the first edition of this book. In that time, I have helped a large number of trainees to construct a Ruth L. Kirschstein training grant. At the same time, my grant-writing seminar expanded from a single, 1-h seminar to an interactive 6-h seminar covered in two, 3-h sessions. Through both of these services, I've interacted with many trainees and their mentors, I've answered questions that may be specific to their situation or may be more general in nature. Regardless, I realized through these questions that there were topics and concerns that I hadn't even considered or that I unintentionally omitted when writing the first edition. Further, some of the questions highlighted the fact that I didn't discuss certain topics in enough detail. Therefore, I felt the need to include these issues and provide clarity in what I had previously written.

More importantly, the National Institutes of Health (NIH) have made several significant changes in the Ruth L. Kirschstein training grant application packet since the first edition of this book was published. Some of these changes involved general topics made to all NIH grant application (e.g., Biosketch), others were changes that specifically applied to these training grants (e.g., submission of References, etc.), and some are newly required sections (i.e., Institutional Environment and Commitment to Training). Regardless of whether these changes or additions were general or specific, they were significant enough that parts of the first edition of this book were obsolete.

In the second edition I have expanded and updated the original version to include all of these topics. Specifically, I describe the combining of previous sections (Doctoral Dissertation and Other Research Experience, Goals for Training, and Activities Planned) into a new section entitled "Applicant's Background and Goals for Fellowship Training." I discuss how an applicant or sponsor's productivity is now illustrated through a new subsection of the Biosketch call "Contributions to Science." I include information on the newly required section "Description of Institutional Environment and Commitment to Training" and where appropriate I provide more detail on how to tailor your writing style to the type of grant you are applying for (i.e., F30, F31, or F32). Further, I highlight the importance of providing a clinical slant to the overall training of MD/PhD students applying for the F30 mechanism.

In addition to these major changes, I also expanded discussions on issues that may be considered minor, but yet are important to consider when constructing a training grant. This information includes updating the process by which References submit their recommendations and providing information on formatting issues to improve the overall visual image of the grant application (i.e., including "white space" and care in the use of acronyms). Finally, through these 5 years I found that many times, trainees had little to no understanding of the basics of the NIH, including the overall structure of the NIH, the common granting mechanisms available through the NIH, and the individuals at the NIH who assist in the review process and the postreview awarding of the applications. Therefore, I have included a brief description of these topics.

I never deluded myself into thinking that my book would become a New York Times bestseller, nor that I would get rich and retire off of the royalties. Honestly, fame and fortune have never been driving factors in my career and life choices that I make. What I set out to do 5 years ago when I sat down to work on the first edition of this book was to write something that I knew was needed, a resource that I knew would educate trainees and mentors on the ins and outs of constructing a training grant, and a guide that I hoped would contribute to trainees being successful in garnering important and prestigious funding. Through word of mouth, from direct interactions with trainees, and from reading reviews of my book on Amazon.com (which my Mom checks on a regular basis!) I know that in that respect I have been successful. It is my sincere hope that this second edition, updated to reflect changes in the Ruth L. Kirschstein grant application package, continues to do what I originally set out to do.

Andrew D. Hollenbach, Ph.D.
January 2018

PREFACE FOR THE FIRST EDITION

There have been two significant experiences in my life that led to me writing the book you have in front of you. First, as a junior faculty member just starting out in my career I had my postdoctoral researcher write a Ruth L. Kirschstein F32 training grant. Ignorant of the extent of information that was required and the overall focus of this type of application, we wrote the grant focusing entirely on the science. I was surprised, and even somewhat put out, at all of the additional sections that needed to be written (including the sponsor information, training plan, applicant information, etc.). Thinking that the F-series grants were similar to the R-series of research grants, we focused mostly on the science and simply wrote something to "fill in the space" for all of the other sections. In our naiveté, we thought we had a strong application and felt that there was no way that we wouldn't get funded. However, we were shocked when the grant came back triaged (the term used in the past for grants that were not discussed). Years later, after sitting on my first F-series study section, which turned out to be a truly eye-opening experience for me, I realized how naïve I had been about the Ruth L. Kirschstein training grants and just how bad the grant was that we had submitted.

Second, in my career there have been several people who truly made a difference in my training as a faculty member and through their help, guidance, and mentoring made it possible for me to advance in my academic career. In particular, there was a colleague and friend at another institute, Dr. Erica Golemis. While I was writing what would become my first successful R01 research grant, she offered to read through what I had written. She had served on multiple study sections and knew exactly what the reviewers were looking for. Further, she was a well-funded investigator and knew what was required to write a successful grant. When she offered to read my first R01 research grant application from the perspective of a reviewer, I enthusiastically took up her offer. However, even at that stage of my career, after having others cursorily read my grants with no real mentoring involved, I was skeptical that I would receive the training and mentoring that I needed, even from a trusted friend and colleague. I was happily proven wrong when she took the time to thoroughly read my grant, constructively criticize what I had written, and then spend hours working closely with me, teaching me how to construct a solid grant. This mentoring and training, for which I am eternally grateful, resulted in my being awarded my first R01 grant, which secured my research, my tenure, and my position in academia.

Since my time serving on the F-series study sections, I have encountered many students and postdoctoral fellows who want to apply for a Ruth L. Kirschstein training grant. Many of these trainees and their mentors are naïve of what is required to construct the best training grant they can possibly put together, as I was myself, and as such have grants returned to them, having not been discussed. The more I saw this happening, the more I realized that I had a unique position from my repeat presence on study section to assist trainees and help them understand the extent of information needed for the application, the purpose of every component of the application, and provide insight into exactly what the reviewers are looking for and the biases and prejudices that exist in the reviewing process. Therefore, the above two experiences in my career inspired me to utilize my insider's perspective on how training grants are reviewed, to pay it forward and assist trainees at my institute to prepare the best grant they could possibly put together.

The more students, postdoctoral fellows, and sponsors heard of my willingness to help them in a constructive manner, the more I realized I needed to develop a method to logically present the nuts and bolts of submitting a Ruth L. Kirschstein training grant. From this realization I developed a seminar to present the information, which saved me having to repeat my "spiel" multiple times to several different individuals in each granting cycle. As part of my seminar I provide handouts of my seminar slides, which tend to be very detailed and are capable of existing as a stand-alone document. At some point I realized that my seminar slides formed the skeleton for what could be a manual or book to be used by anyone, not just at my institute, to understand what is required in a Ruth L. Kirschstein training grant and the human bias and opinions that go into reviewing these grants.

In this book, I provide a small biography of Ruth L. Kirschstein and her legacy, I discuss the review process and many of the biases that affect this process, along with providing a detailed description of the purpose of each component of the grant, what reviewers are looking for in each section of the grant, and suggestions for how to concisely and clearly sell yourself and your training potential. It is not meant to serve as the "key to writing a winning grant." Given the natural biases and influences of human nature in the review process, I truly believe that no magic bullet exists to write the perfect grant. However, what I hopefully provide is an understanding of the process and the philosophy behind each component that will allow you to construct the best grant application that you can, with respect to your own history and unique situation.

Andrew D. Hollenbach, Ph.D.
July 2013

ACKNOWLEDGMENTS

I am greatly indebted to the National Institutes of Health publication *Always There: The Remarkable Life of Ruth Lillian Kirschstein, MD* by Alison F. Davis, PhD. This outstanding book served as the primary source for the brief biography of Ruth L. Kirschstein provided in Chapter 1, Ruth L. Kirschstein—The Woman and Her Legacy.

Ruth L. Kirschstein—The Woman and Her Legacy

1.1 RUTH L. KIRSCHSTEIN—A BRIEF BIOGRAPHY

The Ruth L. Kirschstein National Research Service Award (NRSA) training grants from the National Institutes of Health (NIH) are one of the most prestigious training awards given to predoctoral students and postdoctoral researchers in the United States. However, very few people actually know who Ruth L. Kirschstein was, what she accomplished in her career, and why these grants serve as her ongoing legacy to scientific training. Ruth Lillian Kirschstein, born in 1926, was the daughter of immigrants fleeing Jewish persecution in Russia whose original name, now forgotten, was changed to Kirschstein by a tired Ellis Island immigration official. She was raised in Brooklyn, the daughter of two teachers who instilled a love of learning in Ruth through constant exposure to education and culture. As a result of the continual discrimination against Jews at the time, her parents encouraged Ruth to pursue her own interests in life, regardless of societal attitudes. Therefore, Ruth never realized or accepted that there was nothing that she could not accomplish once she set her mind to it. This familial environment also instilled high personal standards of excellence in Ruth. Although classically trained and accomplished in playing the French horn, she realized that her talent was limited and would not allow her to achieve the level of professional excellence that she desired. Therefore, she decided to follow her second love and pursue a career in medicine.

Ruth enrolled in Long Island University in 1943 and after completing college in 1947 applied to medical schools across the country. During this process, she fought gender and ethnic discrimination as a Jewish female, a bias that further exasperated the difficulty of being accepted into medical schools because of the quota system for admitting Jews to professional training programs. Not accepting defeat, she persevered and was finally accepted and enrolled at Tulane University

A Practical Guide to Writing a Ruth L. Kirschstein NRSA Grant. DOI: https://doi.org/10.1016/B978-0-12-815336-9.00001-6

Medical School in New Orleans, Louisiana, becoming the only student from her Long Island University graduating class to be accepted into medical school. In a class of 109 new medical students, Ruth was one of only 10 women and the only Jewish female enrolled that year. She fully dedicated herself to becoming a doctor, eventually becoming interested in the study of disease and the effects of disease on the human body, which ultimately directed her to a career in pathology.

After completing medical school, Ruth elected to perform her year-long internship in medicine and surgery at Kings County Hospital in Brooklyn, New York. This decision was made partly so that she could be near her new husband, Al Rabson, who was pursuing his own internship in New York, but also partly because of Kings County Hospital's humanitarian mission. Kings County Hospital was, and still is, dedicated to providing care to all people regardless of their ability to pay, an attention to social justice that appealed to Ruth and influenced her entire career. During her internship, she was exposed to diseases and infections of all kinds, including tuberculosis, which she contracted and laid dormant in her for years. More importantly, this time in her career exposed her to many different aspects of medicine, training her to become adept at making on-the-spot decisions. A residency in pathology at Providence Hospital in Detroit followed Ruth's internship until her husband was accepted into the pathology residency program in New Orleans. When Tulane University invited her to continue her pathology training, Ruth accepted.

A year later, in 1955, Ruth and her husband moved from New Orleans to Bethesda, Maryland, where Al accepted a research position in the National Cancer Institute (NCI) and Ruth completed a second year of pathology residency. Despite balancing work, home, and a newborn son, Ruth maintained a positive attitude and an incredible enthusiasm, serving as an excellent parent and role model for their son. At this time Ruth also began fighting for the rights of those commonly discriminated against. Her parents had always stressed and enforced the importance of social justice in their children, an awareness that was later influenced by Franklin D. Roosevelt's fireside chats in which he made a call to help those in need. Further, her firsthand experience of racial segregation in the Deep South emboldened her desire to fight against the inequity of segregation and discrimination. Ruth brought this desire with her to the NIH where she fought for pay rises for deserving women and minorities in a system and at a time when these merit-based increases were not common.

During her residency, in addition to her clinical duties, Ruth would sometimes perform research studies with her husband. She had the chance to test out new instruments, such as the Coulter counter, which was invented at the NIH and is now a standard in hospital and cell biological laboratories. Further, in the mid- to late-1950s at the NIH, she was surrounded by a rich scientific environment in what was an exciting time in science. Marshall Nirenberg, PhD, who cracked the genetic code while at the NIH, had an apartment in the same building as Ruth and Al on the NIH campus. She also saw the development of the shift in cancer treatment from the standard of surgery and radiation to the newly-evolving method now known as chemotherapy, in particular, the successful treatment of cancer with methotrexate.

After completing her residency, Ruth accepted a job with the NIH Division of Biologics Standards (DBS). As a "free-floating" pathologist, working with scientists in the NCI and the National Institute of Arthritis and Metabolic Disease (NIAMD), Ruth sought out and developed true collaborations where scientists worked *with* each other instead of *for* each other. In this collaborative capacity, as with many aspects of her career, Ruth demanded a great attention to detail. This is illustrated by the fact that despite a strong interest in studying the link between viruses and cancer, she refused to allow her name to be included as an author on the now-classic paper by Sarah Stewart, MD, PhD, and Bernice Eddy, PhD, in which they established the link between the SV-40 virus and animal tumors. This refusal to be included as an author on a seminal work derived from the fact that she felt not enough attention to detail had been used in the study. This absolute reliance on accuracy would pay off in her later work where she developed ultimate safety in the worldwide use of the polio vaccine.

Growing up in the mid-20th century, Ruth had firsthand knowledge of the fear engendered in the general population by polio, a fear that lasted until 1955 when Jonas Salk's injectable polio vaccine was declared safe and effective. However, soon after the release of the vaccine, two batches generated from the same company were tainted with infectious virus, resulting in 40,000 illnesses, 50 cases of paralysis, and 5 deaths. It was determined that the cause was the unrealized incomplete inactivation of the virus by the method being used at the time to create a "safe" vaccine. To address this issue, the NIH developed a committee to develop new methods of inactivating the virus and hired Ruth to perform safety testing on the resulting vaccine. Tapping into her attention to detail, she developed the most effective and reproducible procedure for testing the safety of the vaccine in animals. Around this time Albert Sabin, MD, developed his oral polio vaccine that utilized an attenuated form of the virus, which had its own potential public health problems. In response to these concerns, the NIH developed a committee to develop standards for determining the safety of new batches of polio vaccine. Once again, through her hard work Ruth developed a method to test the safety of the vaccine in a manner that was reliable and reproducible. She taught this method to manufacturers around the world, subsequently becoming the standard by which all produced lots of polio vaccine were tested for safety.

As a result of the excellent work performed on vaccine safety, Ruth was named the chief of the DBS Laboratory of Pathology in 1965, a mere 8 years after joining the division. As the chief, she was known for her evenhanded management of individuals and for her treating everyone with respect. She was known as an excellent mentor, being nurturing yet allowing her trainees and employees to shine on their own. She also recognized talent and nurtured it, especially when that talent was present in a minority individual. Her energy and enthusiasm for science was a major draw for all who worked for her and inspired many to work hard and dedicate themselves to protecting public health. This leadership style led her group to develop safety tests for other viruses and vaccines, such as hepatitis B; work that led to future vaccine development.

In 1972, the DBS was transferred from the NIH to the Food and Drug Administration (FDA), where Ruth was made deputy associate commissioner for science. Immersing herself in the position, she learned all aspects associated with the job, including law, bureaucracy (and how to avoid being snared in it), and administrative finesse; all talents that would serve her well in her future career. After one and a half years, she applied for, interviewed, and in 1974 successfully became, the first female director of an NIH institute, the National Institute of General Medical Sciences (NIGMS). As director, she staffed the institute with highly qualified individuals whom she insured for quality by interviewing personally. She developed a team who could effectively balance smart decision-making, team play, and hard work, thereby increasing morale at the institute, which ultimately strengthened the NIGMS. She was involved in all aspects of the institute, almost to the point of micromanaging. However, by bringing her great attention to detail to an administrative position, she was acutely aware of everything that happened within all levels of the institute.

As director, Ruth understood that basic research does not necessarily rely on a specific outcome but instead on the results from a growth of knowledge through incremental advances essential for progress. Up until her tenure as director, money for basic research and money for research training, in the form of the NRSA, were separate entities. However, Ruth felt that these two programs should be integrated because the combination of training and research would ensure the long-term support of both. Further, she developed solid relations with politicians on Capitol Hill through her persistence and honesty. She had an uncanny ability to describe difficult concepts in clear terms and to relate the necessity for funding by relating health issues to the personal lives of senators and representatives. As a result of her hard work, the NIGMS budget quadrupled during her tenure.

Soon after starting her position as director, Ruth was asked to chair an NIH committee whose goal was to evaluate the grant peer-review process. She recognized that the process was prone to human error and natural human bias and that the system needed revamping to provide protections from both. Further, she noted the "incestuous" nature of selecting reviewers, in which a reviewer nominated a replacement when they rotated off. This, combined with gender and ethnic biases in the review process resulted in a system that contained few women and few minorities. Her year-long study developed policies that she introduced and are still in place today, changes were made that included members self-nominating for inclusion on a review panel, applicants being allowed to see the critiques from their review, and allowing applicants to argue their case if they believe an unfair or biased critique was given.

Ruth also worked hard to diversify the NIH and examined the programs that targeted underrepresented minorities. She noted that the diversity program at the time, Minority Access to Research Careers

(MARC), while being a solid program, didn't do enough to fully address the issues and only affected a small number of minorities at a handful of institutions. From this realization she developed a new program, the Honors Undergraduate Research Program (HURP), which became a component of MARC. In this program, a series of science honors classes and summer research programs could be implemented at minority institutions to pique interest in science and science careers. Within 10 years of implementing this program, 76% of the program trainees had enrolled in graduate or professional schools. Further, and more generally, Ruth believed that the quality of training depended on its symbiosis with research; and that by investing in training, either to pique an interest in minorities or to support the training of professional school students, the future of science would be strengthened. By being such a strong proponent of training, Ruth was honored in 2002 by having her name added to the NIH's main training program, which thereafter was known as the Ruth L. Kirschstein NRSA training grants.

In addition to fighting for women and minorities in employment and in education, she also fought to change the way people thought about these populations, particularly women, from a scientific and medical standpoint. She knew that science upheld the fact that women and men were not necessarily the same in terms of clinical responses to treatment or even the health issues they dealt with. However, at the time women, by law, were excluded from clinical trials. Through her work, she became the driving force behind changing the laws about the inclusion of women in clinical studies, raised awareness about the importance of addressing men and women differently in terms of medical and clinical issues, and was instrumental in developing what would become the Office of Research on Women's Health.

As director of the NIGMS, Ruth oversaw many programs and initiatives that are widely known today. She formed the Recombinant DNA Risk Assessment Committee whose task was to develop guidelines for recombinant DNA research. The results of this committee revolutionized this field producing research that resulted in several Nobel Prizes. She oversaw the development of a database of DNA sequences, which eventually became GenBank, and after years helped develop this program into the National Center for Biotechnology Information (NCBI). She also assisted in working to develop policies that became the Human Genome Project in 1990, a project whose goal was to sequence the entire human genome. She even became a subject in a clinical trial for combination chemotherapy and multimodal treatment when she was diagnosed with inflammatory breast cancer, a treatment that saved her life and is commonly used today.

In 1993, she became the acting director of the NIH while Harold Varmus awaited his approval by Congress. When Varmus took over the reins, Ruth left the NIGMS to become deputy director of the NIH. In this capacity she worked with Varmus, not always agreeing with his opinions, but working hard to make his visions reality and to truly transform the NIH. During this time, too, as science moved fast in many different avenues, Ruth and Varmus worked hard to explain science and its relevance to politicians, the media, and the population at large. Her position as deputy director continued until 2000, when Varmus left the NIH and Ruth once again became the acting director. During her subsequent 2-year tenure she saw the completion of the Human Genome Project, the development of ClinicalTrials.gov, a database where volunteers could search for ongoing medical studies, the establishment of the National Center on Minority Health and Health Disparities, the creation of the National Institute of Biomedical Imaging and Bioengineering, the establishment (in accord with a new law by President George W. Bush) of the NIH Guidelines for Research Using Human Embryonic Stem Cells, and supported the creation of the Biomedical Research Infrastructure Network, a program aimed at broadening the geographic distribution of NIH funds. Attesting to her true leadership abilities, she led the NIH through the terrorist attacks of September 11, 2001, and oversaw the transformation of the NIH security in response to that tragedy.

After stepping down as acting director, Ruth stayed on at the NIH serving as senior advisor to the new director, Elias Zerhouni, MD. She continued to work at the NIH until her death at age 83 in 2009, a death that occurred as she wished: With her family by her side, at a place that she loved, the NIH Clinical Center. Ruth L. Kirschstein was a truly amazing person. Her life experiences, growing up the child of Jewish immigrants, both of whom were teachers who instilled an attitude of achieving whatever you put your mind to, along with the attention to social responsibility, created a sense of justice and determination that allowed her to persist through any challenges and accomplish great things. She made an impact on everything she did as a clinician, a scientist, and an administrator; addressing issues of public health, health disparities, inequities in science, and creating many aspects of the NIH that are thriving programs today. Most importantly, she was a teacher, mentor, and advisor to many. Ruth loved to harness peoples' passions, tapping into those passions to develop unnoticed talents through her mentoring and nurturing. She was a tough mentor, but fair and caring, just like the teacher in school who pushed you to your limits because they saw what you were capable of even when you couldn't see it for yourself. People were always the main focus for her and she loved the role of teacher. Finally, she believed strongly that providing excellent training to young scientists was the way to ensure the future of scientific endeavors, something she worked tirelessly to provide and ultimately creating one of her many enduring legacies, the Ruth L. Kirschstein NRSA training grants.

1.2 THE LEGACY—THE RUTH L. KIRSCHSTEIN NRSA GRANTS

The overall goal of the NIH Ruth L. Kirschstein NRSA training grants is "to help ensure that a diverse pool of highly trained scientists is available in appropriate scientific disciplines to address the nation's biomedical, behavioral, and clinical research needs." Full information with links to the parent funding announcements for these awards are available on the NIH web site "F-Kiosk—NRSA Individual Fellowship Funding Opportunities" (https://researchtraining.nih.gov/programs/fellowships). There are presently five categories of NRSA awards, each of which addresses a different stage or type of training.

1.2.1 F30—Individual Predoctoral MD/PhD and Other Dual Doctoral Degree Fellows

The purpose of the F30 award is to support individual predoctoral MD/PhD and other dual degree candidates with the goal that this training will increase the number of physician scientists in basic, translational, and clinical research. Physician scientists play an important role in basic biomedical, translational, clinical, behavioral, epidemiologic, prevention, and services research.

1.2.2 F31—Individual Predoctoral Fellows

The purpose of the F31 award is to provide support for promising doctoral candidates who will be performing dissertation research and training in scientific health-related fields relevant to the missions of the participating NIH institutes. The award will provide up to 5 years of support for training leading to the PhD or equivalent degree.

1.2.3 F31 Diversity—Individual Predoctoral Fellowships to Promote Diversity in Health-Related Research

The purpose of the F31 Diversity award is to provide up to 5 years of support for research training leading to the PhD or equivalent degree or the combined MD/PhD degree. These awards differ from the F30 and F31 in that they are meant to provide opportunities for underrepresented minority groups, thereby enhancing the diversity of the biomedical fields. These groups include underrepresented racial and ethnic minorities (including African American, Hispanic, Native American, and United States Pacific Islanders), individuals with disabilities, and individuals from socially, culturally, economically, or educationally disadvantaged backgrounds.

1.2.4 F32—Individual Postdoctoral Fellowships

The purpose of the F32 award is to provide support to promising postdoctoral applicants who have the potential to become productive and successful independent research investigators.

1.2.5 F33—Individual Senior Fellows

The purpose of the F33 award is to provide senior fellowship support to experienced scientists who wish to make major changes in the direction of their research careers or who wish to broaden their scientific background by acquiring new research capabilities as independent research investigators.

As with any NIH award, these grants are available for US citizens only. It is important to note, too, that not all NIH institutes and centers participate in the Ruth L. Kirschstein NRSA program. The participating institutes are listed on the parent funding announcement for each of the individual awards and have links that will provide more information for special requirements that may be in place of the different institutes.

CHAPTER 2

The People Behind the Curtain—Understanding the Review Process

2.1 THE NATIONAL INSTITUTES OF HEALTH (NIH)

Almost everyone in academic science has heard of the NIH, as have many people in the United States. In the world of academic research, receiving funding from the NIH is considered the epitome of obtaining money for many investigators and institutions. However, many trainees, while having heard of the NIH, may not know how the institute is structured or what different types of funding mechanisms are available. The NIH, located in Bethesda, Maryland, is the broad overarching conglomerate of federal research institutes responsible for biomedical and health related research and falls under the control of the Department of Health and Human Services (DHHS). Although some people may mistakenly think that the NIH is a single entity, it is in fact made up of 27 individual institutes and centers that focus on research related to a variety of different disciplines in biomedical science (see Table 2.1).

Individual institutes within the NIH accept most types of grant applications, which can be either solicited or unsolicited. Solicited applications are submitted only in response to a specific Request for Application (RFA) and usually involve a more focused research area that addresses a specific subarea of interest or research within an institute. These RFAs many times derive from money that has been budgeted within an institute to cover research targeting a very specific or focused topic or disease. In contrast, the unsolicited applications do not adhere to a specific announcement, may be submitted at any of the cycle deadlines, and can investigate any area of research as long as the focus of the project falls under the umbrella of a particular institute.

A Practical Guide to Writing a Ruth L. Kirschstein NRSA Grant. DOI: https://doi.org/10.1016/B978-0-12-815336-9.00002-8

Table 2.1 Individual Institutes and Centers Within the NIH
Institutes of the NIH
National Cancer Institute (NCI)
National Institute of Allergy and Infectious Diseases (NIAID)
National Institute of Dental and Craniofacial Research (NIDCR)
National Institute of Diabetes and Digestive and Kidney Diseases (NIDDK)
National Heart, Lung, and Blood Institute (NHLBI)
National Institute of Mental Health (NIMH)
National Institute of Neurological Disorders and Stroke (NINDS)
National Institute of Child Health and Human Development (NICHD)
National Institute of General Medical Sciences (NIGMS)
National Eye Institute (NEI)
National Institute of Environmental Health Sciences (NIEHS)
National Institute on Alcohol Abuse and Alcoholism (NIAAA)
National Institute on Drug Abuse (NIDA)
National Institute on Aging (NIA)
National Institute of Arthritis and Musculoskeletal and Skin Diseases (NIAMS)
National Institute of Nursing Research (NINR)
National Institute on Deafness and Other Communication Disorders (NDCD)
National Human Genome Research Institute (NIGRI)
National Institute of Biomedical Imaging and Bioengineering (NIBIB)
National Institute on Minority Health and Health Disparities (NIMHD)
Centers of the NIH
Center for Scientific Review (CSR)
National Center for Advancing Translational Sciences (NCATS)
Center for Information Technology (CIT)
John E. Fogarty International Center (FIC)
National Center for Complementary and Integrative Health (NCCIH)
National Center for Medical Rehabilitation Research (NCMR)
National Center for Research Resources (NCRR)

In addition to the Ruth L. Kirschstein training grants, which are the focus of this book, the NIH also has multiple different mechanisms of grant support for a variety of different purposes:

Individual Research Grants (R-series):

- **R01 Research Project Grant:** These grants are in many ways the "Holy Grail" of research funding. This mechanism supports a discrete, specified project that will be performed in the lab of the named investigator and will provide up to $250,000/year for up to 5 years.

- *R21 Exploratory/Developmental Research Grant:* These grants support exploratory or developmental research by providing support for the early and/or conceptual stages of project development. These grants are 2 years in duration and provide up to $275,000 for the length of the funding period.
- *R03 Small Grant Program:* These grants support small research projects that can be carried out in a short time period with limited resources and provide $50,000/year for up to two years.

Program Project/Core Grants (P-series):

- *P01 Research Program Project Grant:* This granting mechanism provides support for an integrated, multiproject research program that involves a number of independent investigators who share knowledge and common resources.
- *P30 Center Core Grant:* These grants support shared resources and facilities for categorical research by a number of investigators from different disciplines who provide a multidisciplinary approach to a joint research effort or from the same discipline to focus on a common research problem.

Pathway to Independence (K99/R00):

- These grants are intended to assist postdoctoral trainees in transitioning to their first independent research position and provide up to 5 years of support for early career investigators. These grants consist of two parts: (1) K99 phase: 1–2 years of support for highly promising postdoctoral researchers, and (2) R00 phase: Support for up to the first 3 years of the independent research career. Transition from the K99 phase to the R00 phase is not automatic and is contingent on having a research position and programmatic review of the K99 phase.

While these are the most prominent and notable granting mechanisms, they are by no means the only ones. This book will focus on the constructing of the F30, F31, F31 Diversity, and F32 Ruth Kirschstein training grants.

2.2 INDIVIDUALS INVOLVED IN GRANT MANAGEMENT

Although many individuals are involved with the construction, submission, review, and management of a grant, there are two key individuals within the NIH who are involved with the direct management of the review process and the post-award project:

- **Scientific Review Officer (SRO):** The SRO is the person who manages the review process for grant applications. They are responsible for analyzing each submission for completeness, recruiting reviewers, managing conflicts of interest, assigning applications for review, attending the review panel (also known as a study section), orienting the members to the operations and policies of the study section, documenting a summary of discussions and recommendations, and preparing the summary statements for the applicants.
- **Program Officer (PO):** The PO manages and advises projects (pre- and post-award) as they relate to the individual institutes' research focus. They are responsible for advising applicants about the appropriateness of a project to an institute's research focus or a specific RFA, making funding recommendations to the institute based on the reviews, overseeing the progress of the funded projects, encouraging and developing new scientific opportunities for applications, and helping develop NIH policy.

2.3 THE REVIEW PROCESS

The process by which NIH applications are reviewed is probably one of the most confusing, unclear, and even sometimes infuriating aspects of the federal granting system for investigators who have submitted their work for consideration. In fact, sometimes trying to get funded, or even receiving a favorable review, can feel like you are trying to hit a moving target, blindfolded, with a gun that does not shoot straight! This fact is particularly true for predoctoral or postdoctoral trainees who are at the beginning of their scientific career and most likely have never written a grant before, let alone experienced receiving reviews for submitted grants, or had the experience of serving on an NIH study section. In fact, many times faculty members themselves who serve as their mentors do not fully understand the review process until they have served on a study section and experienced firsthand the discussions, biases, and in some cases outright prejudices that exist as decisions on the quality of a grant are being made. An understanding of how the review process works, the natural human bias and prejudices that come into play, and the circumstances under which individual reviewers may be evaluating the applications, can provide invaluable information to a trainee to assist them in writing the best application that they possibly can.

One of the first things essential for an applicant to understand is that unlike the R-series of research grants (R01, R21, and R03), in which the applications are sent to and reviewed by a study section convened by a specific institute (e.g., the NCI or the NIGMS), the Ruth L. Kirschstein NRSA training grants are, in the majority of cases, reviewed by an interdisciplinary group. There are 20 different interdisciplinary study sections that consist of recurring special emphasis panels with each of these study sections having a different scientific focus (For a complete list see https://public.csr.nih.gov/StudySections/Fellowship/Pages/default.aspx). The members of these study sections are *ad hoc*, meaning they do not hold permanent reviewer status on this study section, and are recruited based on their scientific expertise and how well that expertise fits within the scientific focus of each individual group. For example, the F08 study section on Genes, Genomes and Genetics reviews those applications that focus on the genetics, genomics, and gene regulation of prokaryotic and eukaryotic systems, while the F07 study section on Immunology reviews applications that are aimed at understanding the role of the immune system in all its different interactions and responses. Because the review is interdisciplinary and not dependent on the institute that will ultimately fund the grant, these members review grants whose research coincides with the scientific focus of each particular study section, with the final funding decisions being made by the appropriate NIH institute.

Within each interdisciplinary study section, the members will evaluate and discuss all five types of F-series training grants (F30, F31, F31 Diversity, F32, and F33). Therefore, each reviewer must be aware of the nature of the training grant they are reviewing (i.e., predoctoral training grant vs. postdoctoral training grant) and evaluate the application accordingly. During study section the applications are separated into the five different fellowship types with each group being discussed as a unit. This means that the F30 applications are usually discussed first, followed by the F31 Diversity, the F31, the F32, and if any have been submitted, the F33 applications. Depending on the number of applications under consideration, all of the grants within each group may be discussed or only $\approx 50\%$ of the grants will be discussed. If, for example, only six F30 applications are under consideration, then all of these grants will be discussed, regardless of the initial impact score, and therefore receive a score. However, in the case of the F32 or F31 applications, which are by far the largest in number and can sometimes have upward of 60–70 applications each, only half will be discussed. The cutoff for which applications will be discussed varies from study section to study section, but usually falls at about the 50% mark. If a grant application is not discussed in study section, it will receive a designation of "Not Discussed" on the final Summary Statement in lieu of a score.

The review process begins with the recruitment of the members for each interdisciplinary study section. The SRO invites approximately 25–30 reviewers for each study section. These reviewers are chosen based on their scientific expertise, which is determined by how well their research focus fits into the scientific topic for that interdisciplinary section. Selecting members based on their research focus provides a panel of investigators who will be well versed in the general topic being reviewed and should therefore be able to provide informed reviews and solid criticisms of each grant. Reviewers are *ad hoc*, meaning that no one person is given a permanent appointment to this review group and must receive an invitation for each new study section. However, people can be invited back repeatedly to serve on a study section. A repeat presence is determined by the SRO and can be dependent on the scientific expertise of the reviewer, the quality of the reviews that the person provides, the contributions that the reviewer makes to discussions, or all of the above.

Once the study section roster is established, conflicts of interest between a study section member and any aspect of the submitted grants must be determined. The SRO will provide all members with a list of the grants to be considered. Each member examines this list to see the name of the applicant, the name of the sponsor, the name of the cosponsor (if appropriate), the names of the people who wrote the letters of recommendation, and at what institute the work is being performed. If a study section member knows the applicant, sponsor, cosponsor, and in some cases the people who wrote the letters of recommendation personally, has worked with any of them in the past, or works at the same institute from which the application derived, that member is considered to be in conflict with the application. The reviewer is then recused from reviewing that application and when that grant is being discussed physically will leave the room so as to not hear the discussion associated with the application.

Once the roster is established and conflicts of interest are determined, the SRO assigns up to 12 grants to each study section member. These assignments are made based on the known scientific expertise of each reviewer with the SRO making all best attempts at providing the best fit between application and reviewer. However, it is important to note, particularly as you write your grant, that frequently, if not always, someone will be reading your grant that is not an expert in your field of research. The person reading your grant may be familiar with the techniques and theories you put forward, but will not have firsthand experience with the exact field in which you are proposing for your research. This means they will be versed enough to critique your logic, evaluate your preliminary data, comment on the validity of the proposed experiments, and agree or disagree with conclusions that you draw. However, they will most likely NOT implicitly understand the details of the field. Therefore, it is important to make the assumption that the person reading your grant knows nothing about the field in which you are writing so that you can write clearly and explicitly. If you do not make this assumption, and write your science so only an expert in the field would understand it, you will receive a lower score than might be expected.

Once the applications are assigned, the reviewers will be designated as Reviewer 1, Reviewer 2, or Reviewer 3. Reviewers 1 and 2 are responsible for providing detailed descriptions of the strengths and weaknesses of each individual review criterion (see below) along with a description of the overall impact and merit of the grant. In contrast, Reviewer 3 is only required to provide a description of the overall impact, although they are strongly encouraged to provide detailed information on all criteria. Further, the reviewers will have a mix of grants (F30, F31 Diversity, F31, F32, or F33) and a mix of new submissions versus resubmissions. It is the responsibility of the reviewer to recognize the type of grant they are reading, be aware if it is a new submission or a resubmission, and be aware of what their reviewer status is, because slightly different criteria are used to evaluate the different types of grants with more extensive information being required based on the reviewer status.

After receiving their assignments the reviewers are given approximately 3–4 weeks to read, review, and critique each of the grants for which they are responsible. While reading the application, the reviewers are asked to evaluate five different primary criteria to arrive at an initial impact score: (1) Fellowship applicant; (2) Sponsors, Collaborators, and Consultants; (3) Research Training Plan; (4) Training Potential; and (5) Environment. Each of these criteria is evaluated on a score of 1–9 according to the definitions supplied to each reviewer by the NIH (Table 2.2).

In addition, if applicable, human subjects, vertebrate animals, and/or biohazards are also incorporated into the overall impact score. If the application is a resubmission, the reviewers are asked to determine how well the applicant addressed the previous comments, which is also a contributing factor to the overall impact score. All of these latter items, while not receiving scores individually, are taken into consideration when determining the overall impact score. Finally, the reviewers examine such nonscored items as Responsible Conduct of Research, Applications from Foreign Organizations, Research Sharing Plan, Select Agents, and appropriateness of the requested budget.

While reading the grant, each reviewer is responsible for writing a critique addressing each of the five main criteria listed above. These critiques are intended to be detailed and to discuss in a constructive manner the strengths and weaknesses of each of these criteria. In addition, the reviewers provide an overall impact statement: A paragraph

Impact	Score	Descriptor	Guidance on Strengths/Weaknesses
High	1	Exceptional	Exceptionally strong with essentially no weakness
	2	Outstanding	Extremely strong with negligible weaknesses
	3	Excellent	Very strong with only some minor weaknesses
Medium	4	Very good	Strong but with numerous minor weaknesses
	5	Good	Strong but with at least one moderate weakness
	6	Satisfactory	Some strengths but also some moderate weaknesses
Low	7	Fair	Some strengths but with at least one major weakness
	8	Marginal	A few strengths and a few major weaknesses
	9	Poor	Very few strengths and numerous major weaknesses

Table 2.2 NIH Scoring Table and Descriptors

Minor weakness: An easily addressable weakness that does not substantially lessen impact. Moderate weakness: A weakness that lessens impact. Major weakness: A weakness that severely limits impact.

in which they describe their opinion on the overall impact of the application, and provide descriptions of what they perceived to be the main score driving issues. It is important to note that the overall impact score is NOT an average of each individual criterion score but instead reflects how each reviewer believes the individual strengths and weaknesses of the application will contribute to provide an overall training experience for the applicant. Therefore, it is possible to have an overall impact score that is either higher (worse) or lower (better) than the sum of its parts.

After the critiques have been submitted the SRO calculates the average of the overall impact scores of the three initial reviewers to determine an *initial impact score*. This initial impact score is used to establish the discussion order for the study section meeting. On the day of the meeting the reviewers receive a sheet with a list of all of the grants listed in the order of discussion. On this list the grants are broken down into the different type of grants (F30, F31 Diversity, F31, F32, or F33) and within each type the grants are ranked from best (lowest score) to worst (highest score) based on their average initial impact score. In addition, these scores help determine which grants will or will not be discussed. For example, as stated above, approximately 50% of the F32 grants are discussed. This means that if 60 F32 grants were submitted, approximately 30 will be discussed.

At the study section meeting, which can occur all in 1 day or be extended to 2 days depending on the number of applications under consideration, the discussion proceeds in the order predetermined by the averaged initial impact scores and follows the same format for each grant being discussed. For each application the chair of the study section will announce if any of the study section members are in conflict, and if so, they will be asked to leave the room for the duration of the discussion. The chair then announces the name of the applicant, the title of the application, and the institute at which the work will be performed. The reviewers are asked to state their overall impact score for the application after which Reviewer 1 provides a brief description of the application, the strengths and weaknesses of each section, and what issues drove their score. Reviewer 2 then adds to the discussion by providing their opinion of strengths and weaknesses and score driving issues. Reviewer 3 also does the same. For Reviewers 2 and 3 it is acceptable for them to state "nothing to add" should their opinions of the application not differ significantly from Reviewer 1. The floor is then opened for discussion where all the members of the study section are given the opportunity to ask questions of the reviewers for clarification of the issues, to ask how heavily the issues contributed to the score, why certain issues weighed more heavily than others, why one reviewer gave a significantly different score from another, etc.

In the days before the Internet, only the three assigned reviewers would have access to the full grant application. The remaining study section members would be provided with the Specific Aims page only. Therefore, decisions were heavily dependent on the quality of the three reviewers' critiques and presentations. However, in today's electronic age, all members of the study section have easy access to every single grant application being discussed. Although discussions are still dependent on the quality of the critiques and presentations by the three reviewers (since they are the only ones who have had time to thoroughly read the full application), any member can easily access the application to verify facts or to read individual sections to draw their own conclusions relating to score driving issues or check and validate facts under discussion.

At the conclusion of the discussion the chair will then ask the reviewers to state their new overall impact score, which may or may not have changed as a result of the discussion. These new impact scores establish a range within which all members of the study section should vote. For example, if the new impact scores are 3, 4, and 5, the range in which all study section members are encouraged to vote is a 3–5. However, based on the discussion, each individual member may choose to vote outside of this range if they feel it is appropriate. After the range is established, the chair will then ask if anyone will be voting outside of the range and all members doing so must indicate that they will be doing so by raising their hand. They are not required to state if they are voting higher (worse) or lower (better), simply that they are voting outside of the range. All study section members enter their scores online and the final score that is sent to the applicant is the average of the scores for all study section members.

This entire process, from the initial introduction of the application to the final entering of scores can take anywhere between 5 min and 15 min depending on the level of agreement that exists between the reviewers, how many questions are asked by other study section members, and the extent of discussion that is required to arrive at a consensus.

It is important to note that the sole function of the study section is to determine a score for each individual application. This score is derived from the strengths and weaknesses of each application and as such reviewers are not allowed to draw comparisons between applications. The reviewers are not allowed to discuss the fundability of the application because their job is to simply weigh the merits of each grant. Funding is then determined by each individual NIH institute that ultimately provides the funding. Each individual institute has different criteria and a different budget for the level of fundability and it is this budget and criteria that determines the pay line cutoff. Therefore, an application with a score of a 29 may be funded through the National Institute on Aging. However, a different grant, also with a score of 29, may not be funded through the National Cancer Institute.

2.4 THE ROLE OF HUMAN NATURE IN THE REVIEW PROCESS

The previous discussion provided a description of the process by which applications are reviewed. In a perfect world, all things would be equal and all applications would be judged by equal standards. However, the reviewers are human and as such basic human nature, and all of the biases, prejudices, and influences (both conscious and unconscious) that go along with human nature, come into play in the review process. One of the influences that can affect the quality of the review given by a member is simple time management. It is essential to remember that serving on a study section is not the sole job, nor the primary job, of the reviewer. They are busy faculty members who are juggling many different roles, including running a lab, mentoring trainees, teaching, and administrative duties. Although they are provided sufficient time to adequately evaluate their grants, many times they will wait until the last minute due to simple procrastination. It is also more likely that due to busy schedules they may not have a choice but to read them at the last minute. They will then be confronted with a short period of time in which to read and evaluate up to 12 grants, each of which averages 50 pages and can take anywhere between 2 h and 4 h to complete. Further, the conditions under which a reviewer may actually be reading your application may not necessarily be optimal. Sitting on study section is not the reviewer's "day job," but something they are paid to do as a service to the NIH, and it is a function that is extracurricular to their normal responsibilities. Therefore, many times reading is done under what Peg AtKisson formerly of the Grant Writers' Seminars and Workshops described as the "2-2-2 Rule."

Imagine you are a reviewer who runs a lab with seven workers. Among these workers are two graduate students who require a lot of time because they are new and inexperienced. You spend a majority of your day with these students, more time than you expected, making you frazzled because you didn't accomplish the work you needed to get done. You get home from work around 6:30 in the evening to your two young children. They've missed you and you want to spend time with them. They need to be fed, and then they don't want to go to bed when they are supposed to. Finally, you get them to bed and they are asleep. Because your nerves are shot you decide to have two glasses of wine to calm down. Once the wine is consumed and your nerves have settled, you sit down to start reviewing your list of grants, probably around 10:30 at night. Obviously these conditions are not necessarily conducive to a reviewer's clarity of thinking. However, although slightly exaggerated, this scenario is not too far off the mark and provides an illustration for the potential state of mind in which a reviewer will evaluate a grant. Under these conditions a person may not necessarily be capable of focusing his/her mind to provide an unbiased evaluation of an application.

Along these lines, a tired reviewer will naturally fall back on their natural inclinations while they evaluate an application. For example, in a Ruth L. Kirschstein training application, the evaluation of the Research Training Plan (the science portion) is meant to focus less on the nature of the science and more on how the proposed scientific plan will contribute to the overall training. However, we as scientists are trained to think about how to develop a logical argument to support a hypothesis, how to provide solid preliminary data to support feasibility, how to describe solid experimental design to address the hypothesis, and to discuss how our results will impact the field. While all of these things contribute to and are indicative of a solid training experience, the nature of reviewers is to focus on these issues for the science itself and not for how the science will provide a solid training. Although this is a very subtle difference in perspective, it can make a significant difference in the evaluation of a training application and how that application will fare in study section.

Another aspect of human nature that greatly affects the review is the fact that people simply have differences in opinion. These differences in opinion can, and do, affect all of the individual criteria under evaluation. Also, because of these differences in opinion, and the biases, personal experiences, and prejudices that contribute to the formation of these opinions, there will be very different viewpoints on what will constitute a solid training potential. Several of these differences in opinion manifest themselves in the following ways.

2.4.1 The Bias of the "Big Name" Sponsor

Investigators who are leaders in their fields have achieved this status through years of hard work and a history of publishing groundbreaking science in highly respected journals. This status usually means that the "big name" sponsor has a reputation that precedes them. Because they are leaders in the field the basic assumption is sometimes made that simply because they have this reputation that every single person trained in their lab is going to get a top-notch training experience. Frequently a comment such as "if they survive that lab of course they're going to get a good training" or "I was blinded by the Nobel Prize" or even "they have a history of developing new techniques so of course this novel technique (with no data to support its feasibility) will be successful" are heard in study section. As such, a generic or brief and uninformative training plan may be tolerated more readily from a "big-named" sponsor, while a similar training plan from a less prestigious or less established sponsor would be critiqued more stringently or harshly. Another way in which this bias may manifest itself is through the fact that the feasibility of an extremely high-risk Research Training Plan may be accepted more readily without preliminary data to support it from the lab of a "big-named" sponsor. Many people on the study section realize, however, that just because a person is an exceptional scientist does not mean they will be an exceptional mentor nor that high-risk science is any more technically feasible in the lab of a "big name" sponsor.

2.4.2 The Bias of the "High-Power Institution"

As with the "big name" sponsor, an application that comes from a "high-power institute" may be given leeway that would not be given to many other applicants. As with the big name sponsors, high-power institutes, such as Johns Hopkins University, Harvard University, the Mayo Clinic, or St. Jude Children's Research Hospital, achieved their reputation through decades of producing top-notch groundbreaking research, being the home of multiple Nobel laureates, or being places that revolutionized education and/or medical technology. Just as described above, descriptions of facilities and environment that are brief and uninformative are tolerated more in applications from high-power institutes. Further, high-risk science and the development of novel techniques are also considered more feasible in the absence of preliminary data than similar quality applications from non-high-powered institutes. However untrue this reality may be, this bias still exists and requires greater attention to detail in the preparation of the application for investigators not in big name labs or at high-power institutes.

2.4.3 Quantity Versus Quality—What Constitutes Solid Applicant Productivity?

Another issue frequently debated during study section is what is considered good productivity for the applicant. This issue may be difficult to determine and is dependent on the type of application being discussed. An applicant for the predoctoral F31 training fellowship who is in their second year of training is not expected to have as many publications as an F31 applicant that is in their fourth year of training. Similarly, a postdoctoral trainee who has just started their fellowship is not expected to have publications from that lab. However, they are expected to have a solid publication record from their graduate work. Regardless, in both cases the issue frequently under discussion is a comparison of the number of publications that an applicant has versus the quality of those publications, which is determined through what I call "the dreaded impact factor."

A journal's impact factor is determined by the average number of citations a journal receives relative to the overall number of papers published in the previous 2-year time period. While a useful rubric, it may not adequately represent the status of a more specialized high-quality journal for a particular field. For example, the journal *Biochemistry* is considered to be the top journal in which to publish for someone working in the field of biochemical research. However, because it is a journal for a more specialized field the number of citations that journal receives would not necessarily be high thereby giving this journal a lower impact factor. Therefore, in study section a publication in *Biochemistry* would not be considered as reputable as a publication in *EMBO Journal*, a journal with a wider scope and readership interest. In these situations, the bias usually exists that between two applicants in which all else is equal; the applicant with three publications in lower impact journals may not necessarily seen to be as productive (nor creating as much of an impact) as an applicant with one publication in *Cell*, *Science*, or *Nature*.

2.4.4 Quantity Versus Quality—What Constitutes a Good Sponsor Training History?

In evaluating the sponsor, reviewers consider their history of training mentees. The sponsor's training history is illustrated through the number of trainees that have graduated from their lab and the positions these trainees subsequently secured upon leaving that lab. In some cases this evaluation is simple. For example, a junior faculty member who has run an independent lab only for a few years and has yet to graduate any students or complete the training of any postdoctoral researchers will not be considered to have an adequate training history. In contrast, a faculty member who has run their lab for 20 years graduated over 20 students who secured postdoctoral positions in excellent labs with subsequent academic faculty positions will be considered to have an exceptional training history.

The difficulties arise when reviewers are confronted with a junior faculty member who has successfully trained a small number of students; however, these students have all proceeded to high-quality positions. Any investigator who has trained multiple students knows firsthand that although you think you knew how to mentor a student when you were just starting out, there are simply aspects of mentoring that can only be learned through experience. However, isn't it also true that a junior faculty member who has trained a few students to exceptional positions has proven their mentoring capabilities? To some reviewers all they see are the numbers. To other reviewers all they see is where the students have gone, but they may consider these exceptional placements as an aspect of the student's excellence and not necessarily an indication of the mentor's capability. Yet some reviewers are capable of realizing that part of the excellence of where the student has gone must certainly derive from the mentoring capacity of the sponsor. Again, these differing considerations result from differences in opinion between what each reviewer believes to be fact, opinions that derive from their individual career experiences.

2.4.5 The Bias of a Large Laboratory Versus a Small Laboratory Environment

One important aspect to be considered when evaluating the training environment is the number of individuals that will be working within the laboratory during the training period. One applicant may be working in a laboratory that only has two students and a laboratory technician or manager while another applicant may be working in a laboratory with seven students, five postdoctoral researchers, and three laboratory technicians. While each of these environments have their strengths and weaknesses, the reviewers many times view these strengths and weaknesses differently. While a small laboratory environment will allow the sponsor to have more hands-on training with the applicant, the small environment may be seen to be not as conducive to interactions that provide additional training experiences. In contrast, a large laboratory environment provides multiple opportunities for the applicant to interact with a variety of people at very different stages in development. However, in that large environment the ability of the sponsor to provide a significant amount of hands-on training with each individual person is significantly called into question. The question then boils down to the issue of what is more important in the training, the access to multiple "mentors" (a large laboratory environment) or the ability of a single mentor to truly shape and mold an individual (a small laboratory environment). As with anything else, the answer to this question is different for each reviewer.

2.4.6 All Strengths and/or Weaknesses Are Not the Same—Impact on Training Potential

Probably the single criterion that is the most subjective in the review process is the training potential of an application. This criterion takes into consideration all of the different aspects of the grant (including the applicant, the sponsor, the science, and the environment) and as such is influenced by all of the biases just described. Because of natural differences in opinion, the extents to which an individual's strengths or weaknesses will contribute to or detract from the training potential are also considered differently. Further, the extent to which a particular strength alleviates the concern of a particular weakness, and vice versa, is also considered differently and may not necessarily be the same for all applications under consideration. Let's examine the situation where an applicant may propose the development of a novel investigative model in their Research Training Plan that is by no means certain of success. Despite the high risk of this model, there is no preliminary data to support the feasibility of this model. Further, all of the experiments in the proposal depend on the success of this model. Assume that this uncertain model was proposed by an applicant who is being trained in a small lab from a junior investigator at a mid-range academic institution. In this case the Research Training Plan will receive a low score, which will subsequently have a large impact on the overall success of the application. In contrast, should this model be proposed by an applicant in a larger lab from a leader in the field at a high-power institution, the question of feasibility of this uncertain model may not even be considered. The Research Training Plan will then receive a good score and will not significantly affect the overall training potential. This example is only one of many that exists, not only for the Research Training Plan, but also for all aspects of the application, and illustrates the importance of natural bias in the review process.

2.4.7 What Constitutes a Major/Minor/Negligible Weakness?

As described above, each of the individual criteria is scored on a scale of 1−9 with each number being characterized by the quantity and nature of weaknesses present in that section. Although the reviewers are provided with this scoring rubric, and explicitly requested by the SRO to hold to this rubric, the nature of a particular weakness is not necessarily evaluated the same by all reviewers. What one reviewer may consider being a negligible weakness, another reviewer may consider being a minor or major weakness. These considerations would then change a score from a 2 (extremely strong with negligible weaknesses) to a 4 (strong but with numerous minor weaknesses) or even a 7 (some strengths but with at least one major weakness). Further complicating this issue is the fact that multiple aspects of an application may contribute to or alleviate the nature of a weakness. In the example above, the presence of the applicant in the lab of a big-named researcher at a high-power institute could alleviate the concern of an unproven model system from a major weakness (giving it a score of 7 or worse) to a minor or possibly even negligible weakness (giving it a score of 4 or better).

The issue over what is considered a minor, moderate, or major weakness is exacerbated even more when determining the score for the overall impact of an application. As stated above, the overall impact score is the opinion of reviewers of how the individual criterion, with their respective strengths and weaknesses, will provide an overall successful training for the applicant. While the combinations of strengths and weaknesses within that section can influence the score of each criterion, the overall impact score is then influenced by how each of these individual sections fit together to provide a description of a solid training potential. In the context of the larger application, a weakness that may have impacted an individual criterion heavily (an untested model system) may not have as much importance in the overall training potential when considered beside the other criterion (sponsor, institute, and applicant). The importance of these strengths and weaknesses are determined by each individual reviewer through the lens of human nature influenced by their own personal experiences and opinions.

2.5 TIMING OF SUBMISSION IS EVERYTHING

There are three submission cycles for NIH grant applications, with each different grant mechanism (i.e., R-series, P-series, F-series, etc.) usually having different timelines for submission, review, financial recommendation, and start date. Within each cycle are key dates including the due date (the absolute deadline for submission), review (when study sections will meet to review the applications), advisory council (the second round of review to recommend funding of scored applications), and start date (when the funding will be made available for use by the investigator). As can be seen in Table 2.3 7–8 months elapse between the date that the application is officially submitted and the date that a successful grant would receive the funding for the training period.

Because of the length of the elapsed time between the official submission of the application and the receipt of funds for a successful grant, trainees have a window in which they may submit and/or resubmit their applications. For example, consider the case where a graduate student at the end of their second year of training will submit an F31 grant application for the August 8 deadline. This application will then be reviewed in October or November in what would be their third year of training. Assuming they receive a fundable score, decisions made on funding would be finalized in January with funds being received by the trainee in April of their third year. In this case, the trainee would have over 2 years of training remaining during the

Table 2.3 Submission Deadlines for the Ruth L. Kirschstein Training Grants			
Due Date	Review	Advisory Council	Start Date
April 8	June/July	October	December
August 8	October/November	January	April
December 8	February/March	May	July

funding period. Even if this application does not receive a fundable score in the first attempt, a driven trainee and sponsor will try to resubmit a revised application for the December 8 deadline. In this case, assuming a successful revision was submitted, the funds would be received in July between their third and fourth year, still providing them with at least 2 years in their training.

Now consider a situation in which a trainee is between their third and fourth years of training wanting to submit an application for the August 8 deadline. Using the timeline above, if successful, the trainee will receive the funds in April of their fourth year of training. If a resubmission of a revised application is required, and the resubmission is successful, the funds would not be received until July between their fourth and fifth years of training. In both of these situations, the reviewers will consider the dates by which the funds would be received, compare them to the time remaining in the training process, and most likely decide that the applicant should be nearing the end of their training and no longer require funding to complete this process.

As with all aspects of the review process and how human nature influences the review, different reviewers will have different realms of experience with how long a training period should last, since different fields may have different lengths of time for training based on the different types of experiments that are being utilized (e.g., research utilizing animal models requires more time than research using a defined in vitro molecular system). Regardless, trainees and sponsors must be attentive to where the applicant is in their training process and the time that will elapse between submission of the application and receipt of funds if the submission was successful.

What the discussion in this chapter highlights is that although there are distinct guidelines, rules, and examples by which each and every grant is expected to be reviewed with an unbiased eye, human nature exists and as such natural bias, and sometimes even downright prejudice, will be introduced into the review process. It is the necessity of the applicant and the sponsor to have a basic understanding that, although not necessarily fair or correct, these biases exist. As such, the applicant and sponsor must critically evaluate their individual situations, make the best attempt at determining how their individual situation may be perceived by a reviewer, and then use this knowledge to construct the best possible grant to sell themselves and their scientific ideas to the reviewers. In essence, be the salesperson that knows their target audience and write to convince that audience.

CHAPTER 3

Who Are You?—The Fellowship Applicant

The Fellowship Applicant section is one of the five major criteria the reviewers use to evaluate the Ruth L. Kirschstein training grant applications. Within this section, there are multiple components that, when considered together, provide the reviewers with an overall impression of the applicant, their goals, and their qualifications. These components include the applicant's previous academic record and scientific productivity, their previous research experience, their goals for the fellowship training and future career, a description of why the applicant selected their sponsor, department and institute, and letters of recommendation. Each of these sections examines a different aspect of the applicant and when taken together presents an overall picture of their attributes and abilities. Further, several of these components provide information that will allow the reviewers to determine whether the training described in the application is truly a departure from previous training experiences. Therefore, to fully sell yourself as an exceptional applicant, regardless of your history and present circumstances, it is important that you understand the function and importance of each component and how each of these components contributes to the overall reviewer evaluation of the applicant.

3.1 THE BIOSKETCH (5 PAGES MAXIMUM)

In the Biosketch, the applicant provides information describing their previous academic record and their scientific productivity. In addition, they provide information, in the form of a Personal Statement, that details how the training described in the application will provide an overall program that is perfect for them as it relates to their individual future career goals and ambitions and their previous training history. The Biosketch is a standard NIH form containing explicit headings detailing the information required, among which are the applicant's name, their eRA Commons name (a "username" provided by the NIH for each individual), educational history, previous positions held, and

A Practical Guide to Writing a Ruth L. Kirschstein NRSA Grant. DOI: https://doi.org/10.1016/B978-0-12-815336-9.00003-X

academic and professional honors. However, unlike a Biosketch written for an R-series research grant, which focuses more on the science, the Biosketch for training grants focuses on training and the qualities of the applicant. Therefore, the NIH Biosketch for a Ruth L. Kirschstein training grant includes a section for the applicant's academic record (i.e., previous grades and test scores). Further, other sections, such as the Personal Statement, are addressed with a focus on the training that will be provided by the overall application instead of describing their qualifications to carry out the proposed research.

3.1.1 Personal Statement

The Personal Statement is the section of the Biosketch in which the applicant provides a description of their goals as a scientist, their previous research experience, and exactly how the plan described in the application will provide them with the best possible training to advance their career. The Personal Statement can be difficult to write, because it is not always entirely clear exactly what information needs to be included. However, it can be viewed, in some respects, as an "abstract" for the entire application. Just as an abstract in a manuscript provides the reader with a summary of research being presented in a paper, the Personal Statement provides a summary of all of the individual components that describe you, the applicant and how the different aspects of the application fit together to form the perfect training environment for you as an individual. Therefore, it is important to include explicit statements describing the goals for your career, your research training up to this point, how this previous training directed you along your present career trajectory, why you selected the mentor(s) (sponsor and cosponsor) you did, how this sponsor and cosponsor will provide you with the training you need to advance your career, how the present environment will enhance your training, and how the educational program at the institute and department will give you the training that fits your personal needs.

It is usually good to begin the Personal Statement with a solid description of your long-term goals: "My long-term research interests involve investigating molecular pathways that contribute to the development of human disease with the goal of establishing an independent research laboratory at an academic institution." It is important that this statement be direct and detailed but yet general enough so as not to be viewed as disingenuous. The reviewers like to see that you have knowledge of your general research interests (e.g., molecular pathways that contribute to human disease) without unrealistically limiting the potential for changing interests as you progress through your career. Follow this statement with a description of how you became interested in research, once again being explicit but not disingenuous or ingratiating. For example, personal statements may sometimes include statements such as the following: "Ever since I was a child and I saw the wonders of nature around me, I knew that I wanted to become a scientist." Although for some people this statement may be true, reviewers will most likely perceive this statement as saccharine and ingratiating. Instead, if there was a personal experience that motivated your career goals, state it explicitly being sure that it is stated factually, but yet with meaning: "While in graduate school, a friend was diagnosed with and succumbed to leukemia. Upon reading about this disease, I found that many forms of leukemia have a defining genetic characteristic of a chromosomal translocation, which produce oncogenic fusion proteins. From that point on I became interested in cancer biology research, in particular cancers that derive from chromosomal translocations."

For some applicants, it may not have necessarily been a defining moment in their personal lives that motivated their career decisions but instead their present path is a culmination of an overall educational process. Regardless of whether the present training trajectory derived from a single moment (as described above) or an overall process, provide a brief description of your academic history. Where did you perform your previous training (undergraduate and/or graduate if appropriate) and how did that experience contribute to forming your present career trajectory. If there was a specific class or teacher that made an impact on your decision to pursue academic science or a particular research focus, you should include that information, but in a reserved and factual manner. It is also important to include a statement that describes the factors driving your decision to choose your present training program and mentor. For example, if you are a graduate student that underwent laboratory rotations, state: "As part of the graduate program at X, I underwent a series of laboratory rotations during my first year of graduate school. Through these rotations, Dr. Y impressed me with her hands-on, nurturing mentoring approach. Further, her research sparked my interest as it relates to my long-term goals." Finally, concisely summarize how the overall training that you will receive is perfect for you: "Taken together, the skills learned from my experience at this institute and completion of the training plan put forth by Dr. Y and the Departmental program, along with ample mentoring opportunities available here, will equip me with the diverse qualities needed to pursue a career as an independent researcher in an academic environment."

Sometimes an applicant may have had issues in their past or present personal situations that may limit or affect the perception reviewers have of the overall quality of the described training plan. These issues may include personal family situations that require an applicant to remain within a specific region or even the same institute to continue their training; personal health issues that caused an applicant to take a hiatus from their training or created a perceived gap in their publication or training history; health or personal issues of a previous mentor that delayed publication of previous work; or even simple immaturity and indecision at an earlier stage of training that resulted in poor academic grades. Regardless of the reason, it is important that these issues be addressed directly, but in a professional manner, in the Personal Statement. Remember, although it may not necessarily seem like it when reading their critiques, the reviewers are human and understand that even though an applicant may have the best intentions, that sometimes life simply gets in the way. Further, it is even more important to remember that reviewers usually read applications very closely and will see inconsistencies in your past (such as a gap in your training). If no reason is given to explain these inconsistencies, the reviewer will "assume the worst" and your overall score will suffer accordingly.

In general, reviewers will respect honesty and openness, as long as it is not perceived as an excuse for poor past performance. Further, it is important that you provide a description of why this past issue is not an impediment to your present and future excellence. For example: "During my undergraduate career I was not entirely sure of my dedication to academics. Because of this indecision I did not perform as well as could be expected in my classes. However, during my junior year when I took a course in X, I discovered my passion for Y and as a result fully applied myself to this newfound love. Now, I am dedicated to realizing my goals of becoming an independent scientist, as illustrated by my significantly improved grades in my final year of undergraduate and in graduate school."

Finally, it is very important to remember to write the Personal Statement keeping in mind the type of training grant for which you are applying. For example, a person applying for the F31 predoctoral grant or the F30 MD/PhD grant is at the beginning of their career training. Therefore, they are at the stage in their development in which they are obtaining the broad base in knowledge, skills, and scientific thought they need to develop into a strong scientist. In contrast, the postdoctoral researcher applying for an F32 fellowship has already obtained this knowledge. Therefore, their training needs to focus on the techniques and skills that are essential for them to transition to an independent academic position, keeping in mind that these skills are not only technical but also include mentoring, presentation, laboratory management, and transitioning to independence. Further, the career goals of the F31 predoctoral applicant (who are training to become academic scientists) are very different from those of the F30 MD/PhD applicant (who are training to become clinicians/scientists) and as such they require a different type of training in order to achieve these goals.

3.1.2 Contributions to Science (Publications)
As with an established investigator on an R-series application, a training applicant's scientific productivity is determined by their list of publications. In the past, an applicant would simply list their publications, with this list being limited to the top 15 articles most relevant to the submitted application. However, more recently, this format was changed to include the section entitled "Contributions to Science". The purpose of this change was an attempt to diminish the effect that the "impact factor" of a publication may have on the reviewers' perception of the importance of the productivity of the applicant. Instead of merely listing the top most relevant articles, it is now the job of the applicant to provide a narrative stating exactly how the work that was performed made a significant contribution to science.

When organizing this section of your Biosketch, each stage of your training path (i.e., undergraduate, graduate, etc.) should be contained within a single paragraph. Within this paragraph provide a brief but descriptive explanation of the work that was performed during this stage of your training, concluding this description by explicitly stating the conclusions that were drawn from your work. Wrap up each paragraph with an explicit statement; "This work is significant because..." and then continue on to state exactly how the conclusions drawn from your work advanced the field of study, how this work established feasibility for subsequent research, or even how this work established a model system or method essential to the lab in which you worked. Once you have stated this significance include the statement "The significance of this work is indicated through the following publications:" at which point you provide your bibliography *as it pertains the work you just described in the associated paragraph* in a bulleted list, adhering to the NIH standards for references.

It is important to note that the information in the "Contributions to Science" section of the Biosketch is very similar in nature to the information that is included in the "Doctoral Dissertation and Other Research Experience" section (to be discussed later). However, there is a distinct and important difference in what the reviewers are evaluating in each section, which requires you to write each of these with a different focus. In the "Doctoral Dissertation and Other Research" section, you need to focus on several different things: (1) Describe how the research you performed in the past provided you with a solid research experience; (2) Illustrate your ability to see a project through to a logical conclusion; and (3) Provide the basis for the reviewers to evaluate whether the work you are proposing in the present application is a significant departure from your past training experiences. In contrast, in the "Contributions to Science" section of the Biosketch, you need to explicitly demonstrate how the work you performed in your previous training was important enough to make a significant contribution to science. In other words, you must illustrate to the reviewers that you are capable of performing what some may consider important research, research that is capable of changing the way people think about a field or how people approach a particular question. The differences in the focus that you provide in the writing of these two sections may seem like subtle differences, but they are very important differences. One focus tells the reviewer that what you did before demonstrates you have the ability to *perform* the research; the other tells the reviewer that the work you perform is capable of *making a noticeable contribution* to your field of study.

Unlike an established investigator who has been working in their field for years or even decades, the applicant for a training grant will not necessarily have an extensive list of peer-reviewed articles. The reviewers understand this fact and recognize that depending on the nature of the grant for which you are applying (i.e., F30/F31 vs. F32) you may or may not have peer-reviewed publications. For example, a second-year postdoctoral fellow applying for an F32 training grant will be expected to have peer-reviewed publications from their graduate work but not necessarily from their present postdoctoral position. Along these same lines, a second- or third-year graduate or MD/PhD student applying for an F31 or F30 will also not necessarily be expected to have any publications from their present graduate training. In both cases, though, having peer-reviewed publications, either from their past work or their present position, will greatly enhance the overall perceived quality of the applicant.

Therefore, it is important to consider several alternative forms in which an applicant can demonstrate their productivity. These alternative forms can include publications that are in revision or have been submitted (listing the journal to which they were submitted: "Manuscript submitted to X") and manuscripts that are in preparation (listing the journal to which you intend to submit: "To be submitted to X"). It is important to note, however, that these types of publication listings *do not carry nearly the weight as an accepted or published manuscript.* The reason they do not carry as much weight is that unless a manuscript has been accepted for publication, it has not endured the rigors of peer review and has not been "validated" by that process. Regardless, these manuscripts in development demonstrate to the reviewers that your work has progressed to a point at which you are able to prepare it for scrutiny by your peers.

It is also acceptable to include published abstracts, poster presentations, and invited talks, including all regional, state, national, and/or international venues in which your work was presented. Although not published in a journal, which indicates to the reviewers and to the scientific community in general that your work passes the scrutiny of review, these last three categories demonstrate that you have been productive enough to have your work recognized on a larger stage and accepted for dissemination to the scientific community. Finally, regardless of the type of publication, it is highly recommended that you use bold font for your name and indicate with an asterisk if you are a co-first author on a publication. By doing this you highlight where your name falls in the author listing (first author, co-first author, middle author, etc.), thereby making it easier for the reviewer to determine your contributions to the work included in that publication.

3.1.3 Scholastic Performance

The scholastic performance of the applicant is illustrated by the grades they achieved throughout their education. The Biosketch form that is provided by the NIH for the Ruth L. Kirschstein training grant has a table for entering academic grades and this table and form must be used. When entering your grades into this table it is important to remember to include ALL of your grades from your undergraduate and graduate institutions and not just your science-related grades. The reviewers want to see the full range of academic capabilities, not simply in the science-related classes. Also, selecting and choosing which grades to present may raise a question to the reviewer that there may not be full disclosure about your academic performance. It is extremely important to clearly delineate which grades come from which institution. Remember, the reviewer may be reading your application under suboptimal conditions (see Chapter 2). Therefore, it is essential to be as clear as possible to avoid potentially annoying a tired reviewer who has to work to figure out your academic history. One good rule of thumb is to place all of the grades from an individual institute into one column with the name of that institute as a heading (Table 3.1).

If the list of grades scrolls to a second page retype the name of the institute within the appropriate column on the new page. If you have taken a course that was not graded on an A−B−C scale, identify how the course was graded (Pass/Fail, Honors/High Pass/Pass, etc.) and what criterion was used to derive the different grade rankings. Finally,

Table 3.1 The Listing of Academic Grades			
The University of Delaware		Johns Hopkins University	
General Chemistry	A	Graduate Biochemistry	B
Organic Chemistry	B	Biophysics	B
Physical Chemistry	C	Molecular Biology	A
Instrumental Analysis	B	Bioorganic Mechanisms	B
German	A	Immunology	A
		Seminar	P
		Anatomy and Physiology	HP

Some courses at Johns Hopkins University are graded on a Pass/Fail basis (P/F). Medical School classes are graded as Honors (H), High Pass (HP), and Pass (P), which correlate to scores of 90%–100%, 80%–90%, and 70%–80%, respectively.

include your GRE or MCAT scores and if you are an MD/PhD student it may even be helpful to include your Step 1 Certification results.

Remember, the reviewers are looking for the cream of the crop. It will be the applicants with 4.0 GPAs, GRE scores or MCAT scores in the top percentiles who are ranked highly in terms of their scholastic performance. If you have an academic history in which you've earned a solid mix of As and Bs you will also be considered an exceptional applicant. One C will raise eyebrows and potentially affect your score while more than one C (or even lower) will significantly affect your score. It is important to remember that this is your history. It is finished and there is nothing you can do to change it. However, you must address this issue directly, which can be done in several different ways. First, the focus of these training grants is to assist in the development of an independent researcher, where capabilities and excellence in the lab many times carry more weight than past academic grades. Therefore, have one or more of your references explicitly state that your academic record does not truly reflect your capabilities in the laboratory. Second, many times an applicant had a poor academic performance due to difficult personal issues or simply because they did not know what they wanted to do with their career. If this is the case, concisely and tactfully describe this issue in the Personal Statement of the Biosketch (see above). The reviewers do not want to know the nitty-gritty details of your personal life. However, if your personal life (e.g., taking care of an ailing family member, working two jobs to pay for school, unexpected health issues) impacted your ability to perform to your optimal capacity, it is essential that the reviewers are aware of this fact. Be certain, too, to point out that those issues are no longer a factor in your life and you have focused on your career goals. Finally, many times an applicant has poor grades in undergraduate but then improves significantly in their graduate work. If this is the case, make an explicit point of this in your Personal Statement. As with the second point, this indicates to the reviewers that you now have your act together and are able to focus your attentions on your present training.

3.2 APPLICANT'S BACKGROUND (6 PAGES MAXIMUM)

Recently the NIH created a new section for the Ruth L. Kirschstein training grants called "Applicant's Background". Although this is a newly created section of the application, the information contained within it is not new and in fact groups together three formerly independent sections of the application package: (1) Doctoral Dissertation and Other Research Experience (formerly entitled Previous Research Experience); (2) Goals for Fellowship Training and Career; and (3) Activities Planned Under This Award. Further, instead of giving an explicit page limitation for each individual component, which when combined was four pages maximum, it expanded this page limit to a six-page maximum for the entire new section. Regardless, the information contained within this section of the application still serves the same purpose; to provide the reviewer with information about your past experiences, how these experiences contributed to your overall goals for your training and future, and how your proposed training will inform the activities you plan to undertake during your training.

3.2.1 Doctoral Dissertation and Other Research

In addition to a solid academic record and good productivity, the reviewers want to see that you have previous research experience. This previous experience covers all of your previous work, including high school science internships, summer research programs, undergraduate research projects, and graduate school rotation projects. It is also necessary to describe your doctoral dissertation research up to your present point of education (if you are a predoctoral or MD/PhD student) or your postdoctoral research to the point at which you are writing the application. This description of research experience serves several purposes in the evaluation of the applicant. First, it shows how much research experience you had before entering your present training position. This information is important because the extent of your previous research experience will indicate how much training you will require in your present position and will also provide a measure for the reviewers to use when evaluating your productivity through publications. Again, remember the type of training plan for which you are writing. While definitely a plus to have experience, extensive research exposure is not as essential for predoctoral and MD/PhD students as it is with postdoctoral researchers, who will have completed a thesis project. Part of the assumption with the predoctoral candidates is that they are in the training program to learn how to perform academic research.

In addition to detailing the extent of your previous research experience, this section will also provide information on the scope and variety of your previous experience. The reviewers use this information to determine not only the breadth of your experience but also how much your present training will be a departure from your previous work. There are instances where the applicant has a fairly extensive research history. However, all of their research is in the same field. For example, an applicant performed undergraduate research examining neurodegeneration using cell culture techniques. They then progressed to their predoctoral work where they did a similar type of research in an identical model system but examining a slightly different molecular mechanism. They then apply for a postdoctoral training grant in which their project is also examining neurodegeneration in a cellular system. While there is nothing wrong with having a very focused knowledge of exactly what type of research interests you, the continuation of a homogenous focus of research throughout your entire training history (i.e., neurodegeneration in a cellular system) will not be perceived as providing any additional training opportunities. In this scenario, it is imperative that you point out in your Personal Statement and Goals sections why you chose to pursue such a focused research interest, which can be perceived as limiting your training potential, and explicitly state how the present training will truly broaden your experience and provide you with novel training opportunities. Further, have your sponsor explicitly state in their training plan (discussed in Chapter 4) how the present program will provide you new training.

The previous scenario is not intended to imply that having a defined research interest is a negative thing. However, it is important to remember that in addition to focusing on the training you will receive, this application also examines the maturity of the applicant. Therefore, having explicit ambitions to work in a specific field requires clearly defined reasons describing why you have this apparent "hyperfocus." Many times reviewers see it as a positive when an applicant does, in fact, have a very clear picture of their research interests and goals and their research experience supports this focused ambition. However, in general what the reviewers are looking for is that you will, in fact, gain new training experiences with the money provided by the training grant. These new experiences can be obtained by working in the same field but in a completely different model system. For example, an applicant is interested in the role of signaling pathways in the development of cancer. They pursued this interest in their predoctoral work using a cellular model system. They have now progressed on to their postdoctoral work where they are working in the same field, but have now moved to an animal model system. Although the research focus is the same, they will obtain invaluable experience working with animals and learning how to relate results found in the animals to what is known in cells. Another example would be a case where an applicant performed extensive undergraduate research examining the effects of alcohol on regulating gene expression in muscle development using a cellular model. Their present dissertation research is now working on the same question in an identical model system. However, instead of examining the molecular mechanisms at work (e.g., transcriptional regulation) they are now using genomics and bioinformatics to look at global gene expression differences and effects. Again, the use of significantly different techniques and cutting edge technology will provide invaluable training in different forms of analysis.

When writing about your previous research experience, it is essential to break down your descriptions into distinct, identifiable sections or paragraphs based on the time period in which you did the work (high school internship, undergraduate honors project, dissertation work, etc.) and the mentor for whom you worked at the time. It is best to present these sections in chronological order from earliest to the most recent. Within each section you need to explicitly describe the research focus of the lab where you worked and what you did during this experience: "The research of Dr. X involves... During my time in this laboratory my project focused on determining..." Tell them how you went about addressing the question of your research and then wrap up the section by explicitly stating the conclusions that you were able to draw from your work; "Through this work I was able to demonstrate that X causes Y, which allowed us to conclude Z." Also, it is extremely important to state whether this work resulted in a peer-reviewed publication, published abstract, or poster presentation in which you were included as an author. "This work was of a significance that allowed my inclusion as an author on..." After you make this statement provide them with a reference, even if that reference is included in your Biosketch. Remember, the reviewer may not want to have to return to your Biosketch to find the reference to which you are referring.

As stated above, the information included within this section is very similar to the information provided in the "Contributions to Science" section of the Biosketch. However, whereas the focus of the writing in the Biosketch needs to inform the reviewer of the *importance and significance* of your previous research, the focus of the writing in this section needs to elucidate *the amount and nature* of your previous experience. In addition to telling the reviewers how much research experience you have and the variety of research training to which you were exposed, this section also demonstrates that you have a history of being able to tackle a project and move it to a logical conclusion at a level that is accepted through peer review or public dissemination.

3.2.2 Goals for Fellowship Training and Career

For an applicant to be considered truly exceptional, not only must they have a solid academic record and history of productivity, but they must also possess a mature and concrete view of their future career plans and they must be able to clearly communicate how the present training will help them achieve these goals. The section "Goals for Fellowship Training and Career" is the section in which the applicant does just that. When stating your career goals it is important to be specific and to clearly state what your career goals are. For example, some applicants will state "My career goal is to run an independent lab in a high-power institute." This statement is vague and tells the reviewer nothing about what field of research inspires and interests you. A better statement would be: "My ultimate career goal is to become an independent researcher at an academic institution and to establish a laboratory that studies molecular pathways that contribute to human disease." While still being somewhat general, it provides a more mature explanation of where you see yourself (an academic institution), what type of research you would like to perform (examining molecular pathways), and what aspect of overall health-related work (human diseases). If possible, it is better to further define the molecular or biological process that interests you and how that process contributes to a more specific health field (e.g., understanding the role of signal transduction pathways in neurodegenerative disease).

Once you have stated your career goals, provide a clear explanation of how the present training and sponsor will help you achieve these goals: "By providing me with extensive training in technical and investigatory aspects related to molecular pathways involved in neurodegenerative disease, this project and sponsor fits perfectly into my future goals of using my research skills to..." Follow this statement by describing the field in which the sponsor works and how that fits your goals, and any explicit technical training that you will receive (e.g., Western blot analysis, DNA isolation, analysis of signal transduction pathways, etc.). It is very important to remember that training does not solely involve the technical aspects of science. Many applications are criticized for not describing the training they will receive in the nontechnical aspects of academic research, which include experimental design, results analysis, manuscript/grant preparation, presentation skills, and networking. These are skills that are essential for a trainee to learn in order to be truly successful as an independent scientist and are usually learned directly from the sponsor. As such, these aspects of training must be explicitly stated. Further, it is important for postdoctoral fellows to describe how the present training and sponsor will help them transition to an independent career and whether they will be allowed to develop a project to take with them to initiate their independent research. It should be noted that the sponsor must also include a similar statement in the Training Plan section of the Sponsor/Co-Sponsor section (see Chapter 4) that confirms that they will, in fact, allow the postdoctoral trainee to take with them to begin their independent career. Along these same lines, applicants for the MD/PhD must detail how the present training will introduce them to the clinical aspects of training that will enable them to become an exceptional clinician-scientist.

Another aspect that must be discussed in this section is the environment in which the training will take place and how the environment will contribute to you achieving your career goals. The environment will provide access to various different resources that will greatly enhance and enrich a training program, including access to cutting-edge technologies, proximity to other institutes to foster collaborations and networking, and journal clubs and/or seminar series that will expose the applicant to invited speakers. Further, if you are a student, it is essential to describe how the Departmental program will provide essential training to obtain your career goals: "The training program set forth by the Department of Genetics will contribute to my long-term goals by providing me with a strong and diverse base of knowledge through a curriculum that includes..." Again, if you are an MD/PhD applicant, you must detail how the MD/PhD program at your institute is perfect for your training goals and how the resources at your institution will enable exposure to clinical-research experiences. Finally, if you are a postdoctoral researcher, it is beneficial to include a description of any career development programs that may be present or what measures your department and/or mentor will take to assist you in a transition to independence. As stated above, it is essential that similar comments appear in the Training Plan section of the Sponsor/Co-Sponsor information attesting to their assistance in helping the postdoctoral trainee transition to independence. Remember, regardless of which training grant you are submitting, you are selling yourself and everything about the training program, which includes the sponsor, the department, the educational program, and the institutional environment. You want to convince the reviewers that as a whole this program is perfect for you to receive an exceptional training. They want to see a multifaceted program that will give you all of the aspects of training that are required to help you achieve a clearly defined long-term career goal.

As with the Personal Statement, it is important to remember the type of training grant for which you are applying. With the postdoctoral F32, the reviewers will want to see a more discretely defined goal than in the predoctoral and/or MD/PhD training grants, because the postdoctoral years are where an investigator truly hones their skills in their field of interest. Also, the postdoctoral researcher is learning the skills needed in order to transition to an independent faculty position. Therefore, it is essential that a description of how the present training will help them achieve that goal of independence (including laboratory management, mentoring, and having a project for them to take with them to establish their independent laboratory) must be included. For example: "Dr. X is dedicated to preparing me for an independent position by teaching me different aspects of laboratory management. Further, through several discussions, Dr. X has agreed to allow me to develop part of my work into a project to take with me to establish an independent lab." This sentiment must then be mirrored and included in the sponsor's Training Plan.

In contrast, reviewers understand that predoctoral students are learning how to think like a scientist and most likely the focus of their doctoral dissertation work will not necessarily be the field in which they work in their independent careers. Therefore, the description of the goals for the present training for predoctoral students should focus more on the training they will receive to think like a scientist and how to develop, analyze, and present their work and be less on the exact field of interest. Finally, when applying for an F30 MD/PhD grant the reviewers usually expect to see a clinical slant in the writing consistent with the potential for clinical and/or translational research in the future. Therefore, the description of the goals for these grant applications must include descriptions on how the training they will receive has clinical aspects involved and how these clinical threads contribute to their overall goals of becoming a clinician-scientist.

3.2.3 Activities Planned Under This Award

The reviewers want to see that you have a distinct and realistic perspective on the time frame in which your training will progress and that the proposed training will be able to be accomplished within the funding period. In the section "Activities Planned Under This Award" you break down each year of your training into a "percent effort" indicating what percent of your time will be dedicated to different aspects of your training. These different aspects of training include research, professional development, teaching/mentoring, and clinical (if appropriate). Present the breakdown of the percent efforts in a table with columns for each of the applicable pursuits and a row for each year of your training (Table 3.2). It is important that you critically evaluate the time you will spend in each of these pursuits, remembering that the primary role of your training is research. Further, the percent efforts should change as the training period progresses. For example, a postdoctoral researcher may have 5% effort in professional development in the first 2 years. However, the final year of training will also involve the search for an independent faculty position, which involves the preparation of your application and going on job interviews. Therefore, your professional development will increase slightly in the final year.

Table 3.2 The Delineation of Activities Planned Under the Award for a Postdoctoral Trainee				
	Research (%)	Professional Development (%)	Teaching/Mentoring (%)	Clinical (%)
Year 1	90	5	5	0
Year 2	90	5	5	0
Year 3	85	10	5	0

The table is followed by a description of what activities you consider to be part of the overall headings. Begin this section with a statement reminding the reviewers that you understand how the training to become an independent investigator involves more than simply the technical aspects of research: "My development into an independent investigator involves undertaking activities not only in the technical aspects of my chosen field but also in the realm of professional development, teaching, and transitioning to independence. Therefore, I will undertake the following activities to achieve my training." While it is not necessary to break down the research into excruciating detail, it is helpful to indicate how long you predict each independent Specific Aim to take to complete. Keep in mind, the reviewers are all investigators and they understand that this is science and a time prediction is just that... a prediction. "I will focus on Experiments 1–3 of Specific Aim 1 in the first 6 months of my training. During this time I will also begin the breeding of mice to generate the animal model system described in Specific Aim 2."

When discussing the professional development aspects of your training, be sure to explicitly and clearly define what you consider to be professional development. Professional development should encompass the writing of manuscripts and grants, presentation of your work, networking, and attendance at seminars and classes important to your education. For postdoctoral fellows, it is essential that the professional development include the learning of laboratory management and the search for an independent faculty position. Finally, the reviewers are expecting that you will progress on to an academic career. Therefore, most study section members like to see that you will have experience in the mentoring of students and possibly limited teaching of classes.

3.3 SELECTION OF SPONSOR AND INSTITUTE (1 PAGE MAXIMUM)

The sponsor, or the mentor/advisor, is the person who has the greatest influence on the direct training of an applicant. As such, the reviewers want to see that the applicant has given careful thought into how they chose this person with whom to conduct their training. Further, the department and institute will also contribute to the overall training of an individual. In the "Selection of Sponsor and Institute" section, you will explicitly and clearly describe why you selected the sponsor, department, and institute in which to perform your training. You need to state exactly what it was about each of these three components that made you feel that this would be the "perfect convergence" of factors to give the best training for you as an individual. In some ways, this section contains similar information as the "Goals for Fellowship Training and Career" section. In both sections you describe how your training will help you achieve your goals. However, while the focus of the Goals section is to talk about how the overall training, which includes the sponsor, department, and institute, *will help you achieve your goals*, the "Selection of Sponsor and Institute" section focuses on the *unique qualities that your advisor, the department, and the institute have that will give you the optimal training you need.*

When writing this section, as with all of the parts of the application, you want to be direct and to the point to make it as easy as possible for the reviewer to see the exceptional nature of your choices and that your selections were mature and well informed. In this section it is also useful to break each of the topics (i.e., institute, department, and sponsor) into their individual paragraphs with each paragraph beginning with a variation of the following "catch phrases." "I chose to pursue my PhD (or MD/PhD or postdoctoral research) at institute X because..." Follow this introductory sentence with explicit reasons for why this institute fits your needs: They have an exceptional educational program that provides a solid basis from which to build your training; they provide diverse research opportunities for a student; they have an interdisciplinary program to enhance your research experiences; a strong collaborative environment exists to promote collaborations, etc. Along these same lines, be very explicit about why you chose a particular department; "I chose to undergo my training in Department Y because..." Again follow this statement with distinct and clear reasons (e.g., the type of research going on in the department, the quality of the research, the supportive caring faculty, the departmental educational program, etc.).

Most importantly, describe your reasons for working with the mentor; "I chose to work with Dr. Z for multiple reasons. Among these are..." When describing your reasons, in particular with your sponsor, remember that the training involves more than just the technical aspects of science. Also it is important to remember that your mentor will be the person who is most influential in your training and will be the one most responsible for molding who you become as a scientist. For many people the mentor–mentee relationship is a personal one, and therefore, in addition to describing how the sponsor's research fits your scientific goals, you must describe how their particular mentoring style is suited for you.

When writing the paragraph about the selection of the sponsor, it may be helpful to think of some of the following questions, determine if these questions apply to you, and if they do, how you would answer them. (1) Does your sponsor have the ability to be more hands-on, which means there will be more extensive interactions between the two of you? This may be important for the predoctoral and/or MD/PhD student who are beginning their training. (2) Does your sponsor take a more distant approach, which means you will be left more to your own devices? This style may be more important for the postdoctoral researcher where independence is required. (3) Does your sponsor have a unique teaching style that has proven results? This is evidenced through the level and quality of career placement that the previous trainees obtained after leaving the laboratory. (4) How does the sponsor teach? Do they use more of a "Socratic" method, which leads you to the question versus a more didactic method, which tells you the answer directly? In addition to thinking about the sponsor and how their mentoring style meshes with how you learn, it is also important to talk about the laboratory environment. Is it a large lab, giving you many opportunities to interact and learn from others? Is it a small lab that creates a closer, more nurturing environment? Finally, after you have discussed all of these characteristics it is essential that you swing it back to focus on you, the trainee, and describe exactly why all of these characteristics that are unique to your sponsor and laboratory environment are perfect for you as an individual and your specific training needs.

Finally, some training grants require that the applicant has a cosponsor or collaborator to supplement the perceived weaknesses of a junior faculty or to provide scientific expertise for a particular aspect of the project (to be discussed in Chapter 4). If you include a cosponsor or collaborator, it is necessary for you to describe why you chose the specific person you did for this role. As with the sponsor description, explicitly state what qualities or expertise the cosponsor will bring. "Because my sponsor is a junior faculty and has limited training experience, I have chosen Dr. X as a cosponsor. Dr. X has a long history of training students and therefore will be able to. . ." However, it is not sufficient to simply pick a cosponsor because they simply "fill a perceived gap" in your sponsor's qualifications. It is important that they also have technical or scientific expertise to complement your project. "In addition, Dr. X has worked in the field of Z for 17 years, as evidenced by his publication record, and will. . ." After this statement, describe how the cosponsor will be instrumental in providing you the training you need as it relates to your project and your career goals. It is also beneficial to mention that the cosponsor will serve on your thesis committee (if you are a predoctoral or MD/PhD student) or on your advisory committee (if you are a postdoctoral fellow). Further, describe how the cosponsor will assist you in experimental design, results analysis, manuscript preparation, etc. What is essential when describing the cosponsor is that their contributions to your training must *seamlessly fit into the overall training plan*. The reviewers want to see that the cosponsor or collaborator will be integral to your training and not simply a tangential figure placed there to "appease" previous critiques or to "pad" your grant application.

3.4 LETTERS OF RECOMMENDATION (3 REFERENCES REQUIRED)

Your letters of recommendation will provide the reviewers with an independent evaluation of your capabilities. These letters also provide a description of a history of excellence, suggesting to the reviewers that this history will translate into a solid potential for your future success as an independent investigator. Therefore, it is essential that you choose the people who will serve as your references carefully. One of the biggest mistakes applicants make is selecting references that all derive from the same institute, if not even the same department, as where the present training is taking place. The department and institute where you are presently working have a vested interest in your success and as such would be expected to write solid letters of support. Therefore, a useful guideline when selecting references is as follows: if you have performed research at another institute (i.e., graduate work, summer internships, undergraduate research, etc.), select your previous mentor to serve as at least one of your references. If you have performed research at several different institutes, then request letters of support from several of these mentors. It is also advisable to select the third reference from within your institute but from a faculty member that is outside of your present department. If possible, make sure that this person serves on your thesis or advisory committee so they are capable of commenting directly on your potential as an independent researcher. It is possible that an applicant, particularly a predoctoral student, may not have performed research as an undergraduate. If this is the case, request a letter of support from a faculty member at the undergraduate institute who is capable of commenting on your potential as an independent researcher. Finally, if you are an MD/PhD student it would be beneficial to get a letter of support from a clinician or someone who can comment on your potential as an independent clinician-scientist, the easiest idea for this being the director of the MD/PhD program. What these guidelines illustrate is the importance of examining your educational and research history and carefully selecting references from each stage of your development to highlight a track record of excellence and a diverse consensus on your abilities as an independent researcher.

When you are deciding on whom to select to serve as references, be sure to select people that you know will write you solid, strong letters of recommendation. This scenario is similar to the adage a defense lawyer takes; never ask a witness a question for which you don't already know the answer. A weak or poorly written letter from a reference will significantly affect how well an applicant will be reviewed. Further, when you contact your references be sure to explicitly ask them to comment on your potential for a successful career as an independent researcher (F31 and F32 applications) or physician scientist (F30 application). If as discussed above you have a poor academic history and this history is not necessarily an indication of your capabilities as a scientist or resulted from external personal issues that were out of your control, select a reference that can explicitly comment on this fact and specifically ask them to discuss this in their letter. For example, an applicant may have had poor grades during several semesters of their undergraduate work. However, their passion was at the bench, where their true capabilities came through, a fact on which the undergraduate mentor can elaborate. Or, if these poor grades resulted from personal tragedy, illness, or unusual circumstances, it is important that the mentor from the undergraduate work makes these facts abundantly clear and explicitly state that the classroom grades in no way represent the true capability of the applicant. Reviewers usually place more weight on the laboratory and scientific skills of the applicant, particularly when references from all aspects of an applicant's training career independently concur on this fact.

The applicant does not submit the letters of reference and more importantly, the applicant is not allowed to see these letters. Instead the applicant must arrange to have the referees submit their recommendations through eRA Commons at the following web address: (https://public.era.nih.gov/commons/public/reference/submitReferenceLetter.do?mode = new). Because the references are being submitted through the eRA Commons and not Grants.gov, the applicant must provide the referees with specific information including their eRA Commons user ID, their last name, and the Funding Opportunity Announcement number. Previously, in addition to the letter of recommendation the referee was required to rate the applicant on a scale of 1−5 for their excellence in a list of 12 individual categories. However, this is no longer the case. Now the referees simply upload a pdf file containing their signed letter of recommendation on letterhead. It is important to note that these references are due by the application deadline and if not received by that time may result in the application being administratively returned without review.

3.5 RESPECTIVE CONTRIBUTIONS (1 PAGE MAXIMUM)

All reviewers know, and expect, that you did not construct this application in a void independent of your sponsor. Further, they realize that your project did not simply materialize independent of the work ongoing in the laboratory in which you are working. Therefore, this section serves as the place where you tell the reviewers exactly what contributions each individual person made to the development of this application and will make in the future work associated with this grant. Some key phrases that may help in the writing of this section are as follows:

- "The development of the research plan put forth in this proposal was developed as a collaboration between Dr. X and myself."
- "The specific aims that will be undertaken derived from small facets of ongoing studies within the lab."

- "This plan was developed from extensive literature research and preliminary data performed by myself."
- "Frequent one-on-one meetings with Dr. X helped me develop this plan."
- "I was responsible for writing the initial draft of this proposal, which then underwent multiple revisions, with the assistance of Dr. X."
- "I will be the primary investigator in accomplishing the work described in this proposal. I will carry out the development of experiments and analysis of results with guidance from Dr. X."

Although this section is probably one of the least scrutinized when evaluating the applicant, it is extremely important that the same care and meticulousness that was used to write all of the other sections be used to write this section, too.

3.6 THE SECOND TIME AROUND—PERFORMING A SECOND POSTDOCTORAL TRAINING

On occasion an applicant who is performing their second postdoctoral training will submit a Ruth L. Kirschstein grant. While this is not necessarily a bad thing in terms of a person's career development, this particular type of applicant will have to provide detailed information describing their reasons for undertaking a second postdoctoral position. It is misguided for an applicant to think that the reviewers will not realize that this is their second postdoctoral experience. The basic fact is that reviewers scrutinize applications for fine details and will in fact notice that an applicant is in their second postdoctoral position and will want to know why a second postdoctoral training period was required. If there is no explicit description, the reviewers may think there is something being hidden from them, which will adversely affect the overall score. There are a multitude of reasons why a person would elect to perform a second postdoctoral training: The applicant's research interests developed in a direction that fell outside the realm of expertise in their present laboratory and they needed additional training; personal issues developed between them and their advisor creating an adverse training environment, etc. However, regardless of the reason, these issues must be addressed either directly or tactfully.

The issue of the second postdoctoral position will need to be addressed in almost every component that relates to describing the applicant. In the Biosketch Personal Statement, be forthcoming with the fact that this is your second postdoctoral position. For example: "During my first postdoctoral training period my research unexpectedly introduced me to field X, which I found to be extremely interesting. Therefore, I decided to perform a second postdoctoral training in this new field to gain more in depth exposure and hands-on experience." Along these lines, this same point must be discussed and expanded in the Goals for Training and Career section, as this is a distinct, and unexpected, change in your career path. Further, this change will also require that you justify the selection of your new sponsor with explicit discussion in the Selection of Sponsor component and a discussion of the research you undertook in your first postdoctoral position in the Previous Research Experience component. Finally, if you left your first postdoctoral position on good terms it is essential for you to have a letter of recommendation from your first postdoctoral advisor, in which that person reiterates why it was essential for you to obtain further postdoctoral training in another lab. However, if the second scenario discussed above, in which you did not leave the first postdoctoral training lab on good terms, is the case, do not include a letter of recommendation from that advisor (as they can not necessarily be counted on to provide you with a solid recommendation) but provide a tactful explanation for this in the Personal Statement of the Biosketch for why their recommendation is not being included. In this latter scenario it is beneficial to also have your present mentor discuss this in their recommendation of you, which is included in the Sponsor's Information section (discussed in Chapter 4).

CHAPTER 4

Who's the Boss?—Sponsor, Collaborators, and Consultants

The sponsor, or the mentor, is probably the most influential person who will be involved in the training of the applicant. Therefore, a detailed description of the sponsor's qualifications as a scientist and as a mentor, along with an explicit outline of the individual training plan they have developed for the applicant, is extremely important for the evaluation of the training potential of an application. Reviewers use several different components to evaluate the overall excellence of a sponsor, including their expertise in the field of study of the applicant's research project, their productivity, their funding history, the number of previous trainees they have produced and the quality of their training, the number of trainees to be supervised during the training period of the applicant, and the training plan for the applicant. As with all aspects of the Ruth L. Kirschstein training grants, it is important to understand the purpose of each of these components in order to convince the reviewers that the chosen sponsor will provide you with the best individualized training possible in order for you to achieve your career goals.

4.1 BIOSKETCH (5 PAGES MAXIMUM)

The sponsor's expertise and productivity in the field of study of the applicant's research project are illustrated through the Biosketch. In general, the sponsor's Biosketch is identical to those used for the R-series research grants (R01, R21, and R03). Just as for the R-series grants, the sponsor needs to provide enough information in the Personal Statement to give the reviewers assurance that they are truly qualified to direct the scientific portion of the application. In addition, it is extremely important for the sponsor to provide information that discusses their dedication to mentoring and teaching and their success in both areas. The dedication of the sponsor to teaching and/or mentoring can be described with examples of their teaching duties, serving

A Practical Guide to Writing a Ruth L. Kirschstein NRSA Grant. DOI: https://doi.org/10.1016/B978-0-12-815336-9.00004-1

on departmental or institutional education committees, etc. The quality or excellence of their mentoring skills, in turn, can be illustrated by using explicit statements that describe where their previous trainees are presently working. For example: "The quality of my mentoring is illustrated through the fact that several of my previous students progressed on to perform their postdoctoral work at top rated institutions, such as Harvard and Stanford Universities." Finally, in addition to supporting the qualification of the sponsor's expertise, their productivity is evident through the number of publications, the topics of these publications, and the quality of these publications, just as described for the applicant (see Chapter 3).

4.2 SPONSOR AND COSPONSOR INFORMATION (6 PAGES MAXIMUM)

Probably the most important part of the application for the sponsor is the section: "Sponsor and Cosponsor Information." In this section, the sponsor provides detailed information about their history and training qualifications, the training environment, and the detailed training plan that they have developed for the applicant. This section is broken down into five parts: Research Support Available; Sponsor's Previous Trainees; Training Plan, Environment, Research Facilities; Number of Fellows/Trainees to be Supervised during the Fellowship; and Applicant's Qualifications and Potential for a Research Career.

4.2.1 Research Support Available

One of the most common questions asked by faculty and trainees who are inexperienced with the submission of these training grants is this: If you are applying for funding to support your training, why does the sponsor have to demonstrate that they have funding in place to support the trainee? What many people do not realize is that the Ruth L. Kirschstein grants will support the trainee's tuition and fees, stipend, and a few thousand dollars a year to cover incidentals (travel, supplies, etc.). Therefore, there are insufficient funds within the award to support the day-to-day research activities of the trainee and their science. The listing of the sponsor's available research support demonstrates that they have money in place, *for the duration of the training period*, to provide the supplies and reagents needed for the successful completion of the research plan.

It is important that you provide information on all present and pending research support. For each of the grants for which you are funded indicate the grant source; the ID number (which tells the reviewers what type of grant you have); the title of the grant; your role on the grant (PI, co-PI, etc.); the dates that the grant is active; and the annual direct costs. This information needs to be presented in a clear, concise, and direct manner, which is most easily done by presenting it in a tabular format (Table 4.1).

If a grant will end during the training period and you have submitted a competitive renewal, this must be stated. If you have a pending grant that has been reviewed and received a solid score, provide this information, too. If you are a junior faculty member and have yet to obtain significant external funding, but are supported through institutional start-up money, this information must be given accompanied by a letter of support from the Department Chair confirming that funds are guaranteed and that these funds are available to support the trainee's research. In general, the reviewers want to see that you have financial support available, or that you are in a solid position to continue funding, for the duration of the applicant's training period.

4.2.2 Sponsor's Previous Fellows/Trainees

Every single person who sits on the study section are themselves established investigators at academic institutions. As a prerequisite to sit on an National Institutes of Health (NIH) study section, these people must have successfully obtained funding from the NIH. Therefore, they are sufficiently senior in their career to have trained a number of students and/or postdoctoral fellows. Because of their own experience, they realize that your ability to train students is an "on the job" learning process and will mature and become fine-tuned with the more trainees you mentor. Granted, some people have the gift of being able to teach and mentor. However, even these gifted people have a level of

Table 4.1 The Presentation of Research Support					
Grant Source	ID Number	Title	PI	Dates	Annual Direct Costs
NIH/NCI	R01CA123456	Mechanism of regulation for the oncogenic transcription factor in melanoma	Smith (PI)	6/01/18–3/31/23	$207,500

naiveté when they begin their independent career that naturally prevents them from being able to provide an optimal mentoring environment. Therefore, the reviewers want to see that you have a history of successfully training people to productive careers at solid academic institutions.

In the "Sponsor's Previous Fellows/Trainees" section, explicitly state the number of previous predoctoral trainees and the number of previous postdoctoral trainees. Do not hide this information in a paragraph that describes your own personal training history. Instead make this information prominent and easy for the reviewer to see:

• Number of previous predoctoral trainees—7
• Number of previous postdoctoral trainees—4

In addition, this section requires that you provide a list of five of your representative previous trainees and describe where they are presently in their career. Telling the reviewer where your trainees progressed in their careers indicates the quality of the training each person received under your guidance. As with the research support, this information is best presented in tabular format where you include the name of the trainee, the years they trained in your lab, their position in the lab, and their current position (including position title and institute) (Table 4.2).

If you have more than five previous trainees, carefully select which of these trainees you list in order to highlight the quality of your training. Further, when selecting which trainees you list, pay attention to

Table 4.2 The Presentation of Previous Trainees			
Name	Years in Training	Position in Lab	Current Position
Alvin Siddy, MD, PhD	2004–09	MD/PhD student	Senior resident in Pediatric Medical Genetics, Detroit Medical Center, Children's Hospital of Michigan, Detroit, MI
Kathy Dent, PhD	2005–10	Graduate student	Postdoctoral researcher, Center for Human Genetics Research, Harvard University, Boston, MA
Mamie Abrigail, PhD	2007–11	Graduate student	Assistant Professor, Department of Zoology, Yale University, New Haven, CT
Kevin Johnson, PhD	2005–09	Postdoctoral researcher	Assistant Professor, Department of Chemistry, Loyola University, Chicago, IL

the type of grant for which your trainee is applying. If they are applying for an F32 postdoctoral fellowship, you will want to list primarily your postdoctoral trainees. If they are applying for an F31 or F30 predoctoral fellowship you will want to primarily list your predoctoral trainees. The reviewers understand that different types of mentoring are required for the different stages of training. Therefore, just because a sponsor has a history of excellence in training predoctoral students, it does not necessarily follow that this person will also be a good mentor to postdoctoral fellows and vice versa. Finally, try to select previous trainees that have stayed within the United States and are presently at academic institutions. While it is not necessarily a major issue that trainees are presently working in foreign countries, the basic line of thought is that these are United States federal tax dollars that are being used to support the training. Whenever a trainee leaves the country it may be implicitly felt, and sometimes even explicitly stated in study section, that federal tax dollars went to support a foreign economy and intellectual environment.

4.2.3 Training Plan

In the Training Plan the sponsor supplies a detailed description of the exact methods to be used to train the applicant. *This plan must be individualized and tailor-made for each applicant.* As stated above, the reviewers have trained their fair share of individuals and realize that every person needs a different style and method of training in order for them to achieve their maximal capabilities. Also, postdoctoral fellows require a different style of training than predoctoral students. Along these same lines MD/PhD predoctoral students need to have a clinical focus in their training, a focus that is not required for a basic science PhD predoctoral trainee. Further, it is important that the training plan does not only focus on the technical aspects of the training but also includes information for the intellectual training and training in nontechnical aspects that a person needs to become a successful investigator. Therefore, one of the most common mistakes a sponsor makes is to provide a generic training plan that gives minimal details and focuses solely on how the research will provide good technical training.

In general, the training plan can be broken down into several different topics: Formal education and examinations (predoctoral students only), technical training, research and professional training, seminars and colloquia, and monitoring of the applicants progress.

Formal education and examinations: While not essential information for the training plan of a predoctoral student, a very short description of the predoctoral or MD/PhD educational program (classes taken, examinations the student will take, etc.) provides information that will indicate a supportive educational environment exists for the training of the student. This information will be covered in extensive detail in the Institutional Environment and Commitment to Training section (covered in Chapter 6), but including an abbreviated version in this section along with the focus on how the formal education will contribute to their overall training is always beneficial. If this information is included, it is important that the Sponsor explicitly state that a more extensive description of the overall educational program can be found in the Institutional Environment and Commitment to Training.

Technical training: Within the training plan the most obvious information to include is a discussion of the technical skills that will be learned during the training period. Many times the first and only thing that a sponsor will discuss in the training plan is the type and extent of technical training that the applicant will receive. However, while technical training is important, it is not necessary for the sponsor to go into too much exhaustive detail about the techniques that the applicant will learn. The reviewers will read the Research Training Plan, in which the scientific project is described, and will be able to evaluate for themselves exactly what technical training the applicant will receive. What is important for the sponsor to discuss in this section is how the techniques the applicant will learn during the present training period *are distinct, different, and new from their previous research experiences and how this new technical training will prepare them for their subsequent career.*

Research and professional training: Oftentimes sponsors neglect to discuss the aspects of training that I refer to as the "intangibles." Unlike the technical training or educational training, where you have a "tangible" outcome in the form of grades or the acquisition of expertise in a new procedure, there are components of training and professional development that do not have such specifically tangible outcomes. These intangibles take many different forms and will be different for the different stages of training and for each individual trainee. A few examples are illustrated through the following questions and suggestions for how to address such "intangibles" in your training plan: (1) How will you teach the applicant to develop a sound project, experimental design, and the analysis of their results? "I will initially discuss the goal of the experiment with the applicant after which I will allow them to design and perform the experiment on their own. I will provide them sufficient time to analyze their results at which time we will meet, the applicant will present the results and their ideas, and I will play Devil's Advocate to discuss the pros and cons of what they did." (2) How will you mentor the applicant in the presentation of their work? "I will discuss the purpose of each section of the manuscript/grant with the applicant, allow them to prepare the first draft, after which I will work closely with them to direct them in the development of a solid document." (3) How often will you meet with them? "Because of my smaller laboratory size, I can give the applicant more personal time and as such I meet with them on a daily basis. In addition, we hold weekly/monthly/periodic lab meetings in which all members of the lab present their work."

In addition to these more direct aspects of training in the experimental and presentational aspects of an independent scientist, it is also important to discuss the educational and teaching components of an academic career. For example, as an academic scientist, the applicant will be required to mentor students of their own and teach in classes, both of which are things that must be learned. Therefore, it is important for the sponsor to discuss within the training plan the opportunities that will be provided for the applicant to gain these types of experiences. These opportunities can take the form of directing a summer or rotation student, assisting in educational outreach programs, or serving as a teaching assistant for a class.

Many times, a topic that is almost never discussed in the training plan, but is important for the ability of the applicant to establish collaborations and to proceed to the next stage of their career, is how will you, the sponsor, provide opportunities for the applicant to network, prepare the applicant for the next stage of their career, and even assist them in obtaining their next scientific position? Several examples for how to address this issue are as follows: "I will frequently discuss the importance of publishing in good quality journals with the applicant"; "The students and postdoctoral fellows are given the opportunity to meet with invited seminar speakers providing them with valuable networking skills"; and "As the applicant nears the completion of their training I will talk about their research interests and assist them in making contacts with colleagues to obtain an appropriate position." What is most important though is in the discussion of these intangibles it is essential for the sponsor to realize that this must be *an individualized plan that is tailor-made for the applicant*. Too many times an application comes to study section in which it is obvious to the reviewers that a "cut-and-paste" approach has been taken. This presents a poor picture on the sponsor and is an indication of the level of interaction and/or attention and quality of training the applicant will receive, or not receive, from the sponsor.

Seminars and journal clubs: It is important that the sponsor discuss the opportunities that will be made available for the applicant to attend seminars on a regular basis. Further, you should mention, if it is the case, that the applicant will have a chance to meet the visiting speaker, which provides invaluable experience in meeting with colleagues and networking to create new connections, collaborators, and/or job possibilities. The reviewers also want to see that the applicant will be given a chance to present their work at departmental, institutional, or regional seminars because it is in these "friendly" environments where they will learn how to effectively present and defend their work. Finally, many reviewers feel that a training plan is not complete without the inclusion of a statement about participation in journal clubs. It is in this educational environment that students and postdoctoral fellows learn how to critically read and evaluate the literature, thereby enhancing their own development and ability to write an effective manuscript.

Monitoring of the applicant's progress: An effective training plan not only needs to contain details of the exact training the applicant will receive but also needs some indication of how the sponsor will monitor the progress of the applicant. This section does not need to be extensive. For example, for predoctoral students this could take several forms, including daily or regular interactions between the sponsor and the applicant, regular thesis committee meetings, or departmental oversight committees. For postdoctoral trainees, in addition to the regular meetings with the sponsor, this could include the formation of an advisory committee that meets on a regular basis.

Inclusion of opportunities to interact with clinicians and/or clinical research (MD/PhD predoctoral students only): The purpose of the MD/PhD training program is to develop the individual into a clinician scientist. This means that in addition to acquiring the basic knowledge and skills needed as a clinician, they also require the skills needed for them to develop and run a viable research program. Many times these trainees have an interest in progressing on to a career in translational science, which marries their two skill sets: Clinical knowledge and basic science abilities. Therefore, it is often beneficial that the Sponsor include information on how the MD/PhD trainee will be exposed to clinical situations or how their thesis project will contain clinical aspects to complement the basic science research. In this way, they will not only get training in how to develop a project and conduct basic science research (the focus of the PhD portion of their degree), but they will also obtain training in how to conduct translational research and correlate basic science findings to clinical situations.

Developing an independent project (postdoctoral fellows only): Every single member of the study section has experienced firsthand the difficulties involved with establishing their first laboratory. They know how critical it is that a postdoctoral trainee has a project that they have developed and are able to take with them to establish their first independent laboratory. Therefore, it is essential that the sponsor include a statement in the Training Plan for a postdoctoral fellow that they will allow the applicant to develop an independent project during their training period to take with them to establish their first lab. Many times the absence of any description that the applicant will be provided with this courtesy, thereby allowing them to "hit the ground running," negatively affects the quality of the training plan and subsequently the overall impact score of an application. It must be noted here that this statement must be mirrored by a similar statement by the applicant in the Selection of Sponsor and Institute section (Chapter 3).

4.2.4 Environment and Research Facilities
The details included within this section of the sponsor's information are also included as a separate section of the application (to be discussed in more depth in Chapter 6). However, even though including

this information in this section may seem to be redundant, the information cannot be abbreviated here. In this component provide information about all aspects of the laboratory, the department, the institute, and the region (if appropriate) that will be supportive of success. In addition to specifics about the laboratory size, proximity to the sponsor's office, etc., this section needs to include information about the proximity to other institutes, any groups that foster interactions/seminars/training, and the intellectual environment of the laboratory and/or department. In the Research Facilities, include descriptions of all required laboratory space, equipment, and any core or animal facilities that are essential to the success of the project and the training.

4.2.5 Number of Fellows/Trainees to be Supervised During the Fellowship

This section of the Sponsor's information is short, sweet, and to the point. Simply list the total number of postdoctoral fellows, predoctoral students, and/or undergraduate students that will be present in the laboratory, and therefore vying for the sponsor's time and attention, during the fellowship period. Also mention any predicted summer students, rotating students or the potential for accepting additional students and/or postdoctoral fellows *throughout the course of the entire training period.* Of course it is not possible for a sponsor to know exactly how many trainees will be passing through the lab for the entire training period; however, it is possible to make a prediction based on past history. For example: "During the period in which the applicant will be in the lab I expect to accept a summer intern each year, two to three rotating students each year, with the potential for one of these rotating students to join the lab."

4.2.6 Applicant's Qualifications and Potential for a Research Career

Simply put, this is the sponsor's letter of recommendation for the applicant. In this section, the sponsor states their opinion of the applicant's capabilities in the tangible scientific and technical aspects and in the "intangible" aspects described above. If the applicant had poor grades as an undergraduate or graduate student, the sponsor can refute this as an issue by telling the reviewers how outstanding they are now and how those grades are not indicative of the applicant's future potential as an independent scientist. If the applicant had personal issues that affected their previous performance or professional issues with a previous advisor that delayed publications, this should be addressed in this section, too. Most importantly, the sponsor must explicitly state their opinion on the potential the applicant has for a successful independent research career.

4.3 IS IT NECESSARY TO INCLUDE A COSPONSOR—YES OR NO?

Probably one of the hardest things to determine, for applicants, sponsors, and even reviewers, is whether the inclusion of a cosponsor is necessary. The purpose of the cosponsor is to contribute qualities to the overall training that may be perceived to be deficient in the primary sponsor. These qualities can include scientific or technical expertise, proven expertise in training, a solid track record of publishing and/or obtaining funding, or all of the above. In some instances the decision to include a cosponsor is not in question. For example, assume the primary sponsor is a junior faculty member who has been in their independent career for only a few years. Because of this junior status, they have yet to successfully train any predoctoral students or postdoctoral fellows, there are no publications from their independent laboratory, and they have a lab with four predoctoral trainees, two postdoctoral trainees, and one lab technician. The lab is still funded from start-up money that will expire in 2 years and this person has yet to obtain substantial extramural funding. From this information it is obvious that this sponsor does not have the requisite training experience, they do not have guaranteed funding for the entire duration of the training period, and in an effort to get as much work done as possible, have taken on a workforce that even a seasoned investigator may have difficulty managing. In this example, a cosponsor who is senior in rank, has successfully trained a significant number of individuals (> 10), has a solid history of funding and publications, and has scientific expertise in the field of the research is required. In contrast, assume the sponsor has been in their independent career for 20 years, has trained 15 predoctoral students and 10 postdoctoral students, the sponsor has had consistent funding for 15 years and they have dedicated funding for another 5, and they have an extensive list of publications in highly respected journals. This person does not need a cosponsor. However, these cases are usually the exception and not the norm.

As a guideline to determine whether you need to include a cosponsor, ask yourself the following questions:

1. Does my sponsor have independent, extramural funding?
2. Does the sponsor's funding cover the entire duration of the training period of the applicant?
3. How many students has the sponsor trained and where have these trainees gone?
4. What is the sponsor's productivity as an independent researcher?

These questions will address many of the issues that reviewers consider when determining the qualifications of the sponsor. If your answer to most if not all of these questions is negative (as in the example given above for the junior investigator), then you should strongly consider including a cosponsor. However, everyone's situation is not necessarily as straightforward as the illustrations given above. For example, a sponsor in mid-career (i.e., Associate Professor in their independent career for 10 years) has funding to cover the duration of the training period of the applicant. However, the sponsor works at a smaller institute and as such has only trained four predoctoral students and one postdoctoral fellow in the 10-year time period. These trainees have gone on to productive careers at such institutes as Harvard and tenure-track faculty at prominent academic institutions. Despite having a small lab size (three individuals maximum at a time) the sponsor has been highly productive publishing an average of one to three manuscripts a year based on research produced in their lab in solid journals for the last 7 years. While on first look it would seem that this sponsor would not require a cosponsor, the reviewers considered the minimal number of students trained as a negative (despite the quality of the training they received) and deemed it necessary for the inclusion of a cosponsor.

Finally, while issues of funding levels and funding duration are very obvious to consider, the issue of training history and productivity are definitely a point of differing opinions among reviewers. In one case, a sponsor may have trained eight predoctoral students and three postdoctoral fellows to outstanding positions in a 9-year career. To one reviewer this may be an exceptional training history, both in quantity and quality. To another reviewer this would be considered a moderate training history and as such score the sponsor lower. Along these same lines, consider the example given above in which the sponsor published one to three manuscripts a year from a small lab. Some reviewers would not necessarily consider this to be a highly productive lab while others would factor in the number of publications and the small laboratory size and deem it to be very productive.

If you find yourself in a situation where you fulfill some of the unstated requirements of what many reviewers consider being a "good" sponsor but not all of them, consider which of the requirements you do fulfill. While reviewers tend to place a heavier emphasis on funding and training history, ultimately it boils down to natural bias in the study section (see Chapter 2). If you find yourself in a "gray area" for a first submission of your application and fulfill some, but not all of these elements, try to sell yourself as a mentor, play up the positives and alleviate the potential concerns the reviewers may have about the negatives, and do not include a cosponsor. If the reviewers then feel that, despite your qualifications in some areas, you still require a cosponsor, include one in the resubmission.

4.3.1 Selection of a Cosponsor

Special care and attention must be made when selecting your cosponsor. In addition to complementing the perceived deficiencies of the sponsor, the cosponsor must provide expertise that is specific to the research project and training of the applicant. In other words, you should not select a cosponsor simply because they have funding or simply because they have trained a large number of people. It is essential that the cosponsor be integral to the training of the applicant, both scientifically and professionally, and to also serve as a "mentor" to the primary sponsor. Further, it is important that the contributions of the cosponsor be *seamlessly incorporated into the entire application*. Therefore, the applicant must provide a description of why they selected this cosponsor (in the Selection of Sponsor and Institute section) and exactly how the cosponsor will contribute to their goals (in the Goals for Fellowship and Career section).

The sponsor must clearly define exactly what the role of the cosponsor will be and the expertise that the cosponsor has that makes them ideal for training the applicant (in the Training Plan section of the Sponsor's Information). For example, describe how the cosponsor will serve on the applicant's thesis or advisory committee; discuss the frequency and forum in which the cosponsor will meet with the student to discuss data and experimental design; and describe any role the cosponsor will play in training of the "intangibles" like manuscript and/or grant preparation and networking. If the applicant is an MD/PhD trainee, it is often beneficial to include a clinician scientist as the cosponsor and have that person be integrally involved with the research project.

Finally, in the Biosketch, which is included along with the Biosketches of the applicant and sponsor, the cosponsor must discuss in the Personal Statement their commitment to mentoring and exactly how they will contribute to the training of the applicant. In addition, the details about the cosponsor's funding status, training history, and number of trainees/fellows to be supervised during the fellowship must also be included alongside this same information from the sponsor. Remember, it is essential that the inclusion of the cosponsor is integral in each and every section of the application, which therefore provides the perception that they are a cohesive and important part of the training experience.

CHAPTER 5

Blind Them With Science—The Research Training Plan

The third major component used to evaluate a Ruth L. Kirschstein training grant is the Research Training Plan, in which you present the scientific project that will be undertaken during the training period. Unlike the R-series of grants, which focus entirely on the quality of the science and the overall experimental design of the project, the Research Training Plan in the Ruth L. Kirschstein training grants focuses more on how the quality of the science, the significance of the project, and logic of the experimental design contribute to the overall training potential. This subtle shift in focus does not mean that less care can, or should, be given to designing the project. A poorly laid out research plan indicates poor mentoring by the sponsor in preparing the application, which indicates a poor potential for training. However, this subtle shift in focus does mean that some things commonly viewed as "fishing expeditions" (such as large-scale genomics screens) are tolerated more in the Research Training Plan than they would be in the R-series of research grants. Despite this "increased" tolerance, these so-called "fishing expeditions" still must be justified by preliminary data or literature evidence and provide evidence that clearly demonstrate a significant contribution to the overall training. Further, although innovation is not explicitly required for the Research Training Plan, the use of what are considered "standard" procedures may detract from the perception of the training potential, unless these "standard" procedures provide the applicant with training in a new field, discipline, or technology.

The Research Training Plan contains all of the components that are present in any standard National Institutes of Health (NIH) research grant *except* for the inclusion of an Innovation section. In general, innovation is not a consideration when evaluating the Research

A Practical Guide to Writing a Ruth L. Kirschstein NRSA Grant. DOI: https://doi.org/10.1016/B978-0-12-815336-9.00005-3

Training Plan. Overall the science portion can be broken down into the following sections:

- Specific Aims (1 page)
- Research Strategy (6 pages)
  - Significance
  - Approach, in which each Aim is broken down into the following sections:
    - Rationale
    - Preliminary Data
    - Experimental Design
    - Expected Outcomes
    - Potential Problems and Alternatives.

The following descriptions are recommendations on how to construct each of the sections for the Research Training Plan. These recommendations derive from a basic understanding of the purpose that each section and subsection plays in the overall grant. The structure and key phrases that are described in the examples below are intended to help focus the writer on the purpose of each section, which should allow you to impart clarity to the reader. It is important to note that the examples that follow are simply recommendations and not intended to be the "perfect" format for writing an exceptional grant. Nor are these recommendations intended to serve as the only way to write a clear, focused, and detailed Research Training Plan. Instead, the following discussion is meant to provide an understanding of the purpose that each section of the Research Training Plan plays in the overall presentation of your project, and to provide key phrases and ideas to help direct your writing while you develop your own writing style.

5.1 SPECIFIC AIMS (1 PAGE)

In the pre-Internet, pre-electronic submission days, the only reviewers that saw the entire grant package for any individual application were the three assigned reviewers of that grant. All of the other study section members received the Project Summary (Abstract) and the Specific Aims page. Therefore, the Specific Aims was the most important part of a science-oriented grant because this was the only part of the application that every member of the study section would have direct access to while discussing the application. Since the advent of the Internet and electronic submission, all study section members, regardless of whether they were assigned the application for full review or not, have immediate access to every single grant under consideration in their study section. Therefore, during study section, instead of simply having the Specific Aims page, each reviewer can quickly and easily pull up an application being discussed to read individual sections, scan the entire document, or just read the Specific Aims or Project Summary. Although the easy access to the entire application in some ways minimizes the original importance of the Specific Aims page, it does not alter the fact that great care must be taken when constructing this section as it serves as a one-page overview of the entire project.

Because the Specific Aims page serves as an overall summary of the scientific project, it must contain all of the elements of the entire Research Training Plan, which includes background of the field, identification of the gap in knowledge, significance of the project, a statement of your hypothesis, literature and preliminary data evidence to support the hypothesis, explicit aims that will address this hypothesis, and how your results will impact the field. Conceptually, the Specific Aims page can be broken down into four sections, which may visually appear as four distinct paragraphs.

Paragraph #1: Conceptually, the first paragraph of the Specific Aims serves as the background and significance. You need to establish the importance of the disease and or scientific question that you are investigating, which is usually established by utilizing statistics of disease mortality or morbidity. Once you establish the health relevance, provide the reader with enough evidence to identify a gap of knowledge in the field. Once you've identified this gap in knowledge, state why it is a problem with advancing of the field, which may include developing effective or novel treatments for the disease state under study. For example: "Although some of the molecular mechanisms regulating the biological activities of the key factors are known, at present the exact role of posttranslational modifications, particularly phosphorylation, in regulating both proteins has yet to be elucidated. The absence of this knowledge will greatly impact the ability to develop novel therapies to treat the disease." Then conclude this paragraph by explicitly stating how the long-term goals of the lab or the explicit goals of your project will address this gap and thereby advance the field: "Therefore, it is *the long-term goal of this lab* to understand how phosphorylation of the key factors regulate their biological activity, how this regulation contributes to normal development, and how this regulation is altered to contribute to the development of the disease."

Paragraph #2: This paragraph is where you describe the objectives of the project and state the central hypothesis of your proposed research. For example: "In keeping with the long-term goals of the lab *the central hypothesis of this project is....*" Follow this statement with a detailed and explicit description of your hypothesis: "...differences in the phosphorylation of the key factors throughout early differentiation contribute to alterations in gene expression, thereby contributing to the development of disease phenotypes." Reviewers like to see what is commonly termed "hypothesis-driven research," in which there is a *very clear and direct hypothesis* that is driving the overall project. Many times a Research Training Plan will suffer because the applicant does not formulate an explicit hypothesis or central driving question or this hypothesis is stated in broad generalities and not detailed specifics.

After the statement of hypothesis, provide a description of the literature evidence that supports this hypothesis: "This hypothesis was formulated from the following literature evidence..." with a concise, yet detailed description, properly referenced, of the literature evidence that supports your hypothesis. In addition to literature evidence, the reviewers also like to see preliminary data that not only supports the hypothesis but also supports the feasibility of the proposed studies. Therefore, state: "In addition to this literature evidence I present preliminary data that further supports the idea that (or provides feasibility for the studies)..." again with a concise, yet detailed description of the data you will present in the Research Training Plan. Finally, wrap up this paragraph by leading into the statement of your specific aims: "We will test our central hypothesis through the following two/three specific aims."

Alternatively, many people start this second paragraph with a description of the literature evidence that they used to develop their central hypothesis. This statement is then followed by a description of the preliminary data that supports the hypothesis and/or the feasibility of the studies. Finally, tie these two different lines of supportive logic together to lead into the statement of your central hypothesis: "Therefore, taken together, this information allows me to propose *the central hypothesis that....*" As with the example above, the statement of the hypothesis leads into the statement of the Specific Aims as described above. It is important to note that bold and italic fonts are purposefully used to highlight the statement of the hypothesis. The use of a different style draws the reader's eye to those words and makes it easy for the reviewer to see that you have a very defined, clearly stated hypothesis driving your work.

Paragraph I section #3: Explicitly state your specific aims in bold letters. This is a 2–3 year project so two to three aims are appropriate. In some cases, a brief one- to two-sentence description of the importance of the aim and the methods that will be used to test the aim can be included:

Specific Aim 1: To examine the role of the phosphorylation of key factors in development and as a contributor to the pathology of the disease. We will use the physiologically relevant primary cells or disease-derived cell lines stably expressing the key factor or mutants in which the identified sites of phosphorylation are mutated to phospho-incompetent or phospho-mimetic amino acids. We will determine how phosphorylation at these sites contributes to normal development and the development of disease by examining cellular functions, such as growth, migration, differentiation, and by performing an unbiased survey to analyze changes in the transcriptome profiles during early myogenesis.

When constructing the specific aims for your project, great care needs to be given to ensure that the aims you are proposing are *interrelated but not interdependent.* What this means is that you want to have all aims contribute to addressing the central hypothesis of your project. However, you don't want the feasibility of one aim to be directly dependent on the success of a prior aim. For example, suppose you propose in Aim 1 to identify and characterize the sites of phosphorylation on a transcription factor. Then in Aim 2 you propose to generate explicit mutants that target the identified sites in order to determine the role they play in biological functions. In this example, although these aims are obviously interrelated, the feasibility of Aim 2 directly depends on the ability of being able to identify the sites of phosphorylation. If you are unable to identify these sites in Aim 1, then Aim 2 is not possible and half of your project is a bust. In contrast, assume you have preliminary data that identifies the only sites of phosphorylation on your protein of interest. Given this knowledge you propose in Aim 1 to determine the effects of these mutations on biological events (e.g., proliferation and differentiation, etc.) and in Aim 2 you propose to determine the effects of these mutants on the molecular activities (e.g., DNA binding, transcriptional activity, expression of target genes, etc.). In this illustration, both aims focus on the effects of the identified sites of phosphorylation have on the molecular and biological functions of the protein. However, the success of the second aim is not dependent on the success of a previous aim.

Paragraph #4: Finally, you want to provide a summary for the reader, which is the conceptual basis of this final paragraph. Tell the reviewer what each aim will achieve and how the successful completion of this aim will provide information that will advance the field: "The research accomplished in Specific Aim 1 will provide an understanding for how changes in the phosphorylation of key factors contributes to both normal differentiation and the development of the disease. Completion of Specific Aim 2 will provide an understanding of the role that phosphorylation plays in regulating the transcriptional and biological activities of the key factors." Also, it is important to tell the reviewer exactly how these results could be used for future studies or what you visualize the long-term impact of this project to be. "Therefore, by understanding the mechanism by which phosphorylation of this protein affects tumor development, we will be able to identify novel molecular targets that can be used for the creation of new pharmaceutical therapies for the treatment of this cancer." Although this scientific program is part of a training plan, the reviewers like to see that you are able to think past the present work and that you understand the potential impact of your results. Many times a grant will not be considered as strong as it possibly could be because the applicant did not adequately demonstrate that they understand the implications of their work to the larger field and future experiments.

It is advisable to include a statement of the contributions that the proposed research will make to the training potential of the individual: "The applicant, an MD/PhD candidate, will develop the necessary technical and critical thinking skills, including the development and analysis of behavioral and molecular studies, to ensure success in a translational research career under the mentorship of the sponsor, an established researcher and MD/PhD scientist in the field of research." Although not essential for a successful application, this final statement summarizes for the reader exactly how the applicant will obtain key training for them to obtain their career goals.

5.2 SIGNIFICANCE (≈ 0.5 PAGES)

In January 2010, the NIH implemented a new, shorter format for grant submissions. This shorter format modified subsections of the grant to provide a different focus than the original, longer form. One of the sections that changed was switching from a "Background and Significance" section to a section entitled "Significance." In the original format the Background and Significance consisted of an extensive, multipage review of the literature that described the field in which the proposed research was being conducted. This section also contained a statement, within the context of the large literature review, of why the research described in the proposal was significant. In the new format, however, the purpose of the Significance section (note the lack of the word Background in the section heading) is to focus entirely on the just that... the significance that the research presented in the Research Training Plan has to impact the field of study. *This section is not intended to replace the Background and Significance section from the old format!* Therefore, the inclusion of a several page discussion of background information is not required, and within the shorter format, which for a Ruth L. Kirschstein NRSA training grant is only six pages for the entire Research Strategy, the luxury of having such an extensive discussion is not feasible.

The purpose of the "Significance" section is to explicitly state why your work is significant in relation to your field of study and how the results from the proposed project will impact the field. The absence of the word "Background" in this new format is not meant to imply that this section does not contain any background information. Background literature is essential to provide the reader with enough context about the field of study so that they can evaluate your interpretation of how the proposed research is significant. In contrast, this background information should encompass only a few sentences and not several paragraphs, or even pages (as was required in the former format). In many respects, this section will provide essentially the same information found in the first paragraph of the Specific Aims page (see above), and in fact it is advisable to paraphrase the first paragraph of the Specific Aims page to begin this section. However, you will provide more detail in the Significance section in discussing the literature evidence that creates the foundation of your proposed work and how your work is essential for advancing the field.

Once you have provided enough evidence to create a solid background foundation, identify the gap in knowledge in the field: "Despite this information, the mechanism by which X does Y to contribute to disease progression is not yet known." Once you have identified the deficiency, explicitly state why this is a problem to advance the field: "Without understanding the mechanism by which X does Y, it will be difficult to develop novel therapies for the treatment of the disease." Then explicitly state in **_bold, underlined, italics_**: "**_Therefore, the contributions of the present proposal are significant because it will be the first study to..._**" As in every other important statement within the Research Training Plan (hypothesis, objective, long-term goals, etc.), be explicit and detailed in your statement. Again, the use of bold, underlined, italics draws the reader's eye and makes it easier for a potentially tired reviewer to see that you have explicitly stated the significance of the work. Finally, as with the Specific Aims, end the Significance section with a statement that informs the reader exactly how the successful completion of the proposed research will push the field forward and could be used for future studies: "By understanding the mechanism by which X does Y we will be able to identify new molecular targets to be used for the development of novel pharmaceutical therapies for the treatment of the disease." As with the Specific Aims, the reviewers like to see that you are able to think past the present project to see the overall implications of the work and that the project is not simply "research for research sake."

5.3 APPROACH ($\approx$ 5.5 PAGES)

The old NIH grant format contained independent sections for Background and Significance, Preliminary Studies, and Research Design. The new, shorter format contains two sections: Significance (which was discussed above) and Approach. Therefore, the background, preliminary data, and research design are all encompassed within the new Approach section, in essence condensing nearly 8–10 pages of writing into an approximately 5-page space. This may at first seem like an insurmountable task. However, the purpose of creating the new format was to help facilitate the review process by decreasing the amount of time a reviewer spent reading an application. Therefore, the new format condenses the writing from a broad-spectrum document to a more focused work that is meant to contain only information that is absolutely essential to support and describe the proposed project.

To condense and focus your writing, it is often beneficial to think of the Approach section in terms of the Specific Aims. What this means is that instead of providing background information and preliminary data *for the entire project*, separate the Approach into parts that correspond to the number of aims that you have proposed and then provide the background information and preliminary data essential *to support that individual specific aim*. Within each section, or specific aim, organize the writing to include three subsections entitled Rationale, Preliminary Data, and Experimental Design. For example, if you are proposing a project with two specific aims, the Approach will be separated into two parts, one part for each aim. The title of each section will be the title of the Specific Aim, *exactly as written on the Specific Aims page*, followed by subheadings for each part:

Specific Aim 1: To examine the role of the phosphorylation of key factors in development and as a contributor to the pathology of the disease.

Rationale: This section includes the *literature evidence* that supports the objective and working hypothesis *for this aim*.

Preliminary Data: This section includes *the preliminary data obtained by the applicant* that supports the hypothesis and the feasibility of the project *for this aim*.

Experimental Design: This section describes the experiments and analyses that you propose to address the working hypothesis *for this aim*. This section also includes a description of the expected results, potential problems, and suggested alternatives should problems arise.

5.3.1 Rationale
About one paragraph in length, the Rationale provides background that supports the working hypothesis *for each individual aim*. It is in

this section that you discuss the *literature evidence* that was used to support the objective of the aim. Much of the same literature evidence mentioned in the first paragraph of the Specific Aims page and in the Significance section will be used in the Rationale. However, the most detail is used here to describe the specifics of the literature. You want to explicitly describe the results in the literature that you have used to support your working hypothesis for this aim. You must provide enough detail such that the reader understands the importance of the results and how the results pertain to the overall objective for this particular aim. However, remember that you have very limited space, so it is important that you be as direct and concise as you possibly can.

Once you have described the literature evidence, summarize what you have just written by explicitly stating how this evidence supports the hypothesis or the feasibility of the aim: "Taken together, this evidence shows that. ..." After this, as with the Specific Aims and the Significance, state what the gap in knowledge is *as it relates to the aim under discussion*: "However, despite this knowledge, the mechanism by which phosphorylation contributes to the molecular mechanisms of disease pathology is not yet known." Follow this statement with a clear and explicit statement of the objective and working hypothesis *for this aim* again written in ***bold, underlined, italics: "Therefore, the objective of this aim is to test the working hypothesis that. ..."***

5.3.2 Preliminary Data

In addition to solid literature support, reviewers almost always want to see preliminary data that supports the hypothesis you have proposed. Through the preliminary data you also give the reviewer confidence that you are technically capable of performing the proposed research and that your model system and/or hypothesis are valid and functional. The validity and functionality of your model system are important. Your training period, regardless of the granting mechanism (F30, F31, or F32), will be about 2–3 years. Therefore, the reviewers do not want to see a proposed project in which you will spend a majority of your time developing or validating a novel model system. They want to see an experimental model in place and know that you are capable of using this model to obtain viable data to address a specific question.

After beginning this section by stating; "In addition to published reports, my preliminary data supports the hypothesis that..."

systematically present *your* preliminary data. If you include unpublished data from another member of the lab, it is essential that you identify this fact. Confusion among the reviewers regarding who actually did the work presented in the Research Training Plan will affect the score of this section and may affect the overall impact score. It is acceptable to include a short statement in the figure legend for a particular piece of data such as: "This data was generated by...." Alternatively, it is also acceptable to include a clarifying phrase in the body of the text when introducing the data in question: "Using data generated by...."

In addition to being clear about who generated the data, it is critical that the inclusion of the figures be presented in an ordered, logical, and neat manner. Many times an application will be submitted in which the figures appear to have been haphazardly imported into the document with no apparent logic for where and how the figures were placed (see Fig. 5.1). Visually this gives the impression of sloppy work and results in a poor first impression, which may suggest to the reviewer that the lack of attention to detail in putting together the application may be indicative of the type of science the applicant will perform or the training that they will receive. Instead, align each figure of data with the paragraph that describes the data, insure that the figures align to the edge of the text, and make sure that there is a consistent distribution of the figures (i.e., all figures align on one side of the page or there is an alteration of alignment) (see Fig. 5.2). Remember, the first impression a reviewer will have is the visual impression. The appearance of sloppy work or a document with no "white space" to provide rest for the eye may predispose a potentially tired reviewer to a negative impression before they even begin to read your science.

When discussing your data, it is recommended to use one paragraph for each experiment, point, or conclusion that you are presenting. This physical and visual separation of experiments allows the reviewer to focus on one thought and idea at a time and gives a visual impression of discrete conceptual units. Also, by devoting one paragraph to each experiment it is easy to import the figure illustrating this data so that it is embedded within the paragraph in which the data is being discussed. The easiest way to import your data into the text is through the utilization of the Text Box tool in Microsoft Word. Simply insert a text box where you would like the figure to appear, copy your data into the text box, and then type the figure number and figure legend

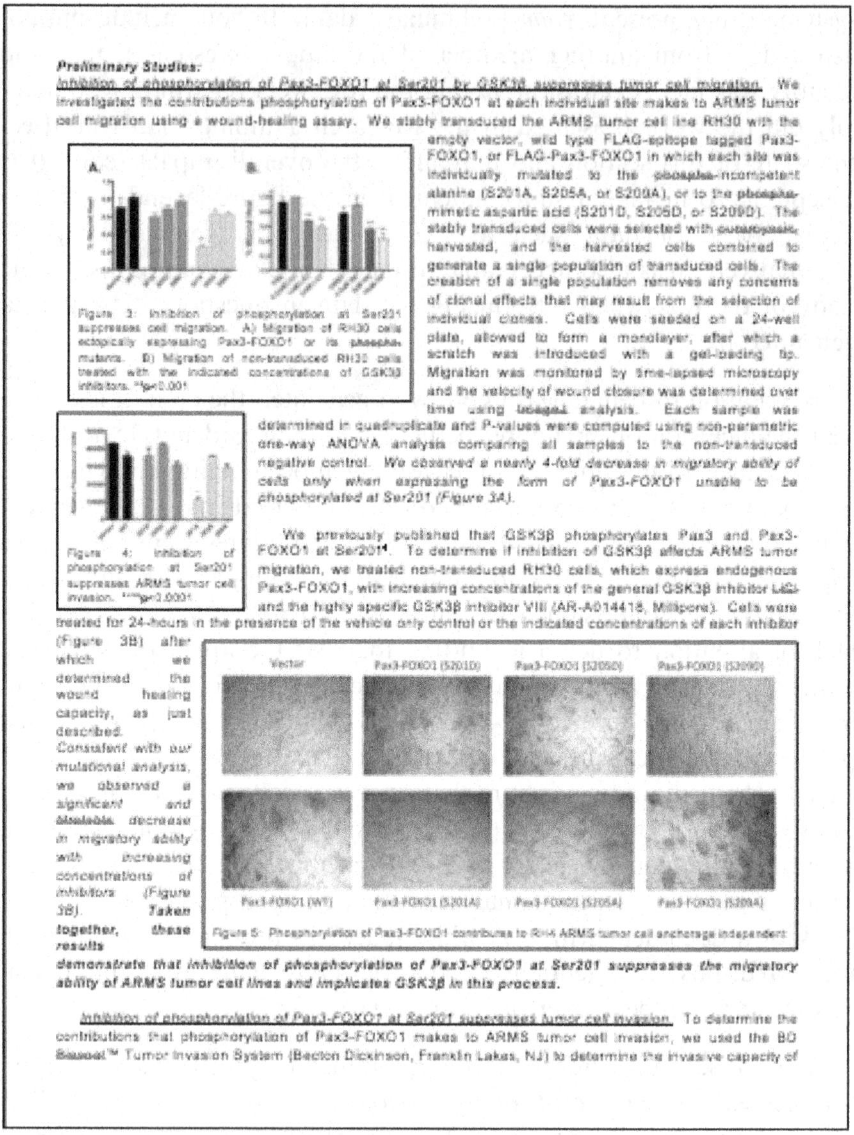

Preliminary Studies:

Inhibition of phosphorylation of Pax3-FOXO1 at Ser201 by GSK3β suppresses tumor cell migration. We investigated the contributions phosphorylation of Pax3-FOXO1 at each individual site makes to ARMS tumor cell migration using a wound-healing assay. We stably transduced the ARMS tumor cell line RH30 with the empty vector, wild type FLAG-epitope tagged Pax3-FOXO1, or FLAG-Pax3-FOXO1 in which each site was individually mutated to the phospho-incompetent alanine (S201A, S205A, or S209A), or to the phospho-mimetic aspartic acid (S201D, S205D, or S209D). The stably transduced cells were selected with puromycin, harvested, and the harvested cells combined to generate a single population of transduced cells. The creation of a single population removes any concerns of clonal effects that may result from the selection of individual clones. Cells were seeded on a 24-well plate, allowed to form a monolayer, after which a scratch was introduced with a gel-loading tip. Migration was monitored by time-lapsed microscopy and the velocity of wound closure was determined over time using ImageJ analysis. Each sample was determined in quadruplicate and P-values were computed using non-parametric one-way ANOVA analysis comparing all samples to the non-transduced negative control. *We observed a nearly 4-fold decrease in migratory ability of cells only when expressing the form of Pax3-FOXO1 unable to be phosphorylated at Ser201 (Figure 3A).*

Figure 3: Inhibition of phosphorylation at Ser201 suppresses cell migration. A) Migration of RH30 cells ectopically expressing Pax3-FOXO1 or its phospho-mutants. B) Migration of non-transduced RH30 cells treated with the indicated concentrations of GSK3β inhibitors. **p<0.001

We previously published that GSK3β phosphorylates Pax3 and Pax3-FOXO1 at Ser201[4]. To determine if inhibition of GSK3β affects ARMS tumor migration, we treated non-transduced RH30 cells, which express endogenous Pax3-FOXO1, with increasing concentrations of the general GSK3β inhibitor LiCl and the highly specific GSK3β inhibitor VIII (AR-A014418, Millipore). Cells were treated for 24-hours in the presence of the vehicle only control or the indicated concentrations of each inhibitor (Figure 3B) after which we determined the wound healing capacity, as just described. *Consistent with our mutational analysis, we observed a significant and titratable decrease in migratory ability with increasing concentrations of inhibitors (Figure 3B). Taken together, these results demonstrate that inhibition of phosphorylation of Pax3-FOXO1 at Ser201 suppresses the migratory ability of ARMS tumor cell lines and implicates GSK3β in this process.*

Figure 4: Inhibition of phosphorylation at Ser201 suppresses ARMS tumor cell invasion. ***p<0.0001

Vector | Pax3-FOXO1 (S201D) | Pax3-FOXO1 (S205D) | Pax3-FOXO1 (S209D)

Pax3-FOXO1 (WT) | Pax3-FOXO1 (S201A) | Pax3-FOXO1 (S205A) | Pax3-FOXO1 (S209A)

Figure 5: Phosphorylation of Pax3-FOXO1 contributes to RH4 ARMS tumor cell anchorage independent

Inhibition of phosphorylation of Pax3-FOXO1 at Ser201 suppresses tumor cell invasion. To determine the contributions that phosphorylation of Pax3-FOXO1 makes to ARMS tumor cell invasion, we used the BD Biocoat™ Tumor Invasion System (Becton Dickinson, Franklin Lakes, NJ) to determine the invasive capacity of

Figure 5.1 Illustration of poor presentation of preliminary data.

immediately below the data *but within the text box.* The inclusion of the figure legend within the text box along with the data it is describing keeps the two items together as a single "unit", which greatly facilitates their positioning and movement within the document. Once inserted simply format the text box so that the body of the text wraps around the box.

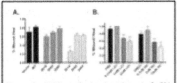

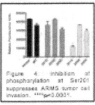

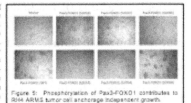

Figure 5.2 Illustration of organized presentation of preliminary data.

In addition, you need to make the basic assumption that the person reading your application will know nothing about your field of research and therefore may not implicitly understand why you performed each experiment or why the results are important to support your hypothesis. It is more than likely that the reviewer reading your grant may be familiar with the techniques you are using, but they will know very little about the field in which you are working. Therefore, you must be explicit, detailed, but yet concise as you describe the thought processes underlying each experiment. In essence, walk the reviewer through each experiment starting with why the experiment was performed, how the experiment was performed, what the results looked like, and the conclusions drawn from these results.

The following rubric can serve as a model for the construction of each individual paragraph of the Preliminary Data section. First, tell the reader exactly what the purpose of the experiment is, how it derived from literature evidence or unpublished data, and how it relates to the hypothesis or model system. "Literature evidence suggests that phosphorylation of the transcription factor is important for regulating differentiation. However, to date, no experiments have been performed to test this idea. Therefore, to determine how phosphorylation at specific sites affects the functions of the transcription factor we tested the ability of different phospho-mutants to alter DNA binding." Once you have established the reason for performing the experiment, provide them with just enough information, usually one to three sentences, to understand how the experiment was performed. This description does not need to include minute details, such as buffers used or concentrations of reagents, but should contain broader strokes that include the experimental system used, the read out that provided the data, and how the data was analyzed.

After discussing the experimental system you next want to describe the results of the experiment. Do not assume that the reviewer will understand or be able to interpret the data simply by looking at your figure! Too many times an applicant will simply write "As evident in Figure X, treatment of cells with the drug inhibits differentiation," without providing an explanation of what the figure is showing, what the control is, what differentiation of this cell type looks like, etc. As stated repeatedly, the reviewer will most likely not be versed in your field of research, let alone be able to interpret data without at least a minimal explanation. Making the assumption that the reader may have an expertise that they might not truly have will only frustrate and anger your reviewer. Therefore, be sure to describe the data to the reader so they can make an intelligent evaluation of the data for themselves. Also, it is important to point out exactly what it is about the results that you want the reviewer to focus on. For example, "We observed the elongation of cells with fusion into multinucleated myotubes, which was confirmed by quantification of the percentage of nuclei present in multinucleated myotubes (Figure X). Further, the presence of the phospho-mutant inhibited differentiation, as evidenced by a decrease in elongation and percentage of multinucleated cells relative to cells expressing the wild-type transcription factor." In general, it is not a good strategy to assume the reader will see exactly what you see in the data or even if they do see it that they will agree with your conclusion if the data is not fully explained to them.

Finally, spell out your conclusions from the experiment and describe why these conclusions are important to support your hypothesis for the aim or to provide feasibility for the experimental model. "This data demonstrates that the ectopic expression of the phospho-mutant inhibits differentiation, supporting the idea that the nonphosphorylated form is essential for differentiation. Therefore, this conclusion supports our hypothesis that. ..." If the data provides feasibility or validity of the new experimental model system, state this fact as follows: "This data demonstrates that we have all of the reagents required for the successful completion of this Aim and that the model system utilized for all experiments is valid to study our working hypothesis." Once you have discussed all of your preliminary data for that specific aim, provide a summary statement to further highlight how, when examined as a whole, the mass of data you presented supports the idea that your project has a high level of feasibility and the hypothesis is sound. "Taken together, published reports combined with our preliminary data demonstrate that the expression of the oncogenic protein results in distinct morphological and biological effects on primary cell differentiation. These observations, which most likely result from global changes in transcriptional regulation, provide solid evidence to support the idea that the presence of the oncogenic protein is capable of altering global transcriptional regulatory networks to result in the observed changes in differentiation, proliferation, and cellular movement." As with other sections of the Research Strategy, the concluding statements for each experiment, along with the overall summary are best written in ***bold, underline, and italics*** to highlight them for the reader.

5.3.3 Experimental Design
After establishing the feasibility of your hypothesis and the validity of your experimental model through literature evidence and preliminary

data, you next logically lay out the series of experiments that you will use to address the working hypothesis of this Aim. As with the Preliminary Data section, each individual experiment will be described in its own paragraph or sentence with the experiments being numbered in sequential order (i.e., Experiment #1, Experiment #2, etc.). Begin each experiment with a descriptive title that tells the reader the purpose of this experiment: "Experiment #1: Determining the effects of phosphorylation of the transcription factor on cellular proliferation." Follow this title with an introductory sentence to tell the reader how this experiment fits into context of the larger scope of the aim: "Literature evidence demonstrates that the transcription factor is involved in multiple aspects of cellular functions, including proliferation. Our preliminary data demonstrates that phosphorylation of the transcription factor contributes to some of these phenotypes. Therefore, this experiment directly tests the role that phosphorylation of the transcription factor plays in cellular proliferation."

After placing the experiment in context, provide several sentences detailing the experimental design itself. As with the Preliminary Data, it is not necessary to provide the minute details of the experiment (i.e., buffer concentrations, reaction volumes, incubation times, etc.). However, it is essential to provide significant details that will allow the reader to evaluate the construction of the experiment and the analysis of the results. This means you should detail the technique that you will be using to perform the experiment. You also need to describe what samples you will use within the experiment and why you are including them, what are the positive and/or negative controls that will be included, what are the time points that will be used (if appropriate), exactly why are you choosing those time points, and what is the output that you will use to determine the results. Finally, you must include a description of how you will analyze the results, reproducibility, and statistics: "To determine how the phospho-mutant alters cellular proliferation, we will compare the results obtained with the mutant to those of cells expressing the wild-type factor. We will perform all experiments in triplicate and normalize values for the negative control of cells not expressing either protein." It is not necessary to discuss the expected results from the analysis at this stage. This information will be provided later in its own section (see below).

One question that arises in the construction of the Experimental Design component of the Research Training Plan is whether a section detailing the exact methods to be used should be included. In the old grant format, where an applicant had fewer space constraints, it was possible to dedicate a full page or even more describing the minutiae of the experimental details in a discrete section dedicated to methods. However, the new format does not allow for such usage of space. The reviewers generally make the assumption that a trainee will be experienced enough to know the details of an individual experiment or if they don't, that they will have the intellectual resources in the laboratory to troubleshoot and learn these details. The reviewers are interested in seeing the "bigger picture" of the experimental design, as described above, and that the applicant understands why they are doing the experiment, what are the essential samples to be used in the experiment, what is the basic assay and read out for the assay, and how will they analyze the results. Therefore, it is usually not recommended to include a specific section of the Experimental Design dedicated to a description of the methods.

5.3.4 Expected Results

To convince the reviewers that you will be capable of interpreting the results of your experiments, you need to provide them with a description of what you expect your results to look like, and how you will interpret them, should your hypothesis be correct. You want to include brief descriptions of the expectations you have for all of the experiments included in the Experimental Design. This section can be difficult to write given the simple fact that sometimes the reason you are doing the experiment in the first place is to determine what will happen. In some cases, you might have preliminary data that will give you very solid groundwork to predict what you will see: "Based on our preliminary data in which the mutation of the transcription factor resulted in an inhibition of the effect, we expect to observe a decrease in our experimental output with our mutant when compared relative to the wild-type control." Sometimes, too, you just don't know what you will see and you have no preliminary data or literature evidence to allow you to make an educated guess. However, you can supply the reader with a *hypothetical* situation that is based on your hypothesis, being very careful to explicitly tell the reader that it is just that... a hypothetical situation: "At present, it is difficult to determine how mutation of the transcription factor will affect cellular biology. However, assuming the *hypothetical* situation in which loss of the site is essential for proliferation, then we would expect to observe a decrease in proliferation rate of the mutant relative to the wild-type control." In essence, you want to prove to the reader that once you get the data and the results from the experiments that you will know how to evaluate them and to interpret them based on your hypothesis.

5.3.5 Potential Problems and Alternatives

Finally, the reviewers want to see that you, the applicant, are aware that problems can, and most likely will exist in the project and that you have alternative methods should you encounter these problems. Remember, if successful, the federal government, through your tax dollars, will be giving you upwards of $100,000–$150,000 in total for your training. They want assurance that if you run into problems that derail your project that this money will not be wasted. Many Research Training Plans suffer from the very simple fact that the applicant did not include any description of potential problems and alternatives to these problems. What is important is that you *do not state that you expect no problems!* This is science. The people reading your application are scientists, many of whom have been working in research for years if not decades. They all know that research is fraught with problems both technical and intellectual. Therefore, the statement that there should be no problems will be viewed for what it is... a naïve statement. However, if there is a technique that you are using that is standard practice in the lab in which you are working you can state the following: "The techniques described in this aim are routinely performed within the lab and as such are not expected to present any major *technical* difficulties." You must be sure to follow this statement up by identifying some valid problems (e.g., transfection efficiencies are inadequate and limits of detection are not feasible) and provide descriptions of viable experimental alternatives to these problems.

Most importantly, unless you have solid evidence that supports your hypothesis incontrovertibly, consider very hard the simple fact that your hypothesis may be wrong. Hypotheses are developed specifically to be tested through experimentation in order to achieve an answer. Part of your training in basic research is to learn that sometimes the answer to these questions are "no" and that your hypothesis as originally constructed is incorrect. Therefore, you must provide the reader with a solid description of what you intend to do should your hypothesis be incorrect, either in part or in its entirety. Are there other pathways that may be considered? Are there other explanations that could lead to the same phenotype that could then be tested? Do you have the ability to reconstruct a new hypothesis on alternative data that can subsequently be tested? Let them see that if your hypothesis is incorrect, that you know what to do, and that you have alternative options or explanations to test so that the money given to you by the federal government will not be wasted. You don't want to undersell or undermine your hypothesis, as that is the cornerstone of your project. However, recognize the fact that hypotheses may not necessarily be correct as constructed.

CHAPTER 6

Last but Not Least: Institutional Environment, Training Potential, and Other Scored Items

There are two remaining major criteria used to evaluate a Ruth L. Kirschstein training grant: the Institutional Environment and the Training Potential. Of these two, the Training Potential is primarily subjective while the Institutional Environment, which is evaluated through three independent sections Facilities and Resources, Equipment, and Institutional Environment and Commitment to Training, is primarily objective. The Institutional Environment has an explicit section in which the applicant and sponsor describe the educational and scientific environment. In contrast, the quality of the Training Potential is determined through consideration of all parts of the grant and how they combine to provide an overall training experience. In addition to these last two explicitly scored criteria, there are several other informational sections that do not receive an independent or *individual* score but whose content contributes to the *overall* score: Activities Planned, Vertebrate Animals, and Research Sharing Plan.

6.1 INSTITUTIONAL ENVIRONMENT

The Institutional Environment is probably the most objective of the five main criteria used to evaluate the application, simply because either the institute has the resources or it does not. The reviewers want to see that the environment in which the training will occur has all of the facilities, equipment, intellectual, and educational resources required to provide the applicant with an optimal training experience. This optimal experience includes easy access to the cores, facilities, equipment, and resources needed to successfully perform the research. In addition to providing explicit descriptions of the facilities and the equipment available to the applicant, it is now required to include an explicit description of the academic, educational, and intellectual environment in which the training will be performed.

Combined, the information that describes the facilities, equipment, resources, and environment is covered in several different places within

A Practical Guide to Writing a Ruth L. Kirschstein NRSA Grant. DOI: https://doi.org/10.1016/B978-0-12-815336-9.00006-5

the application. First, the applicant provides two distinct parts: "Facilities and Resources" and "Equipment," each of which is its own self-contained document and is uploaded separately on the application form. Second, the applicant is required to include an attachment explicitly titled "Institutional Environment and Commitment to Training," which was recently deemed a required document for all applications. Finally, the sponsor includes a description of the training environment within the Sponsor and Cosponsor Information section. In the context of the sponsor's information, the descriptions may not be as detailed, but will in many ways duplicate what is included in the other two sections.

6.1.1 Facilities and Resources

In essence, the reviewers want to see that the applicant has all of the required facilities and resources at their disposal to facilitate the research and the intellectual training. Therefore, the description of the facilities is not to be limited to the physical resources but also needs to discuss the intellectual resources available that will truly enhance the training experience. It is easiest to present this information as explicit sections:

- *Laboratory space:* Describe in detail the laboratory space available. Include a description of the square footage, the number of desks and benches available, and how many people it can comfortably accommodate. If you describe tissue culture experiments in your Research Training Plan, provide a description of the tissue culture facilities and if they are in a separate laboratory, describe the size of this laboratory and the proximity to the main lab.
- *Animal facilities:* If you include animal work in your Research Training Plan, it is essential that you provide a description of the animal facilities at your institute. Tell the reviewers how many rooms are available to the laboratory and the proximity of the animal facilities to the main laboratory. Describe environmental controls (light/dark cycles, temperature, etc.) that the animals will be housed in, especially if these environmental factors are essential to experiments described in the Research Strategy.
- *Office space:* Provide a description of the sponsor's office space, including the square footage and the proximity of this office to the laboratory. If the institute or department provides a graduate student and/or postdoctoral office area, describe this area, include its proximity to the laboratory, and mention how this "communal"

area facilitates interactions between students and postdoctoral fellows.

- **Computers:** Describe the computers that are available in the laboratory and whether each person will have their own computer (desktop or laptop) or whether these computers will be shared. Also, include a statement about what programs will be on the computers that are essential for the work (Microsoft Word, PowerPoint, Excel, graphing programs, etc.) and the connectivity to the Internet.

- **Core facilities:** If your Research Training Plan includes a technique or series of experiments that is perceived to be specialized and therefore requires a specifically trained individual (e.g., genomics, bioinformatics, proteomics, etc.), then describe the core facility that will aid you in these experiments. If a particular instrument is being used in the core, describe that instrument (e.g., Illumina Genome Analyzer 2X with associated equipment for the cluster generation). Indicate, too, who will operate the machine and the training they have.

- **Other resources:** These are resources that contribute to the intellectual development and provide support services to make day-to-day working possible.

  - *Intellectual and training environment:* Provide information on any research or seminar groups to which you belong. Describe any interactions that your lab or department has with other labs or departments in the institute, indicating how these interactions will promote an exposure to different research disciplines. If your institute is in close proximity to other research institutes then discuss this fact and describe any opportunities you will have to interact with these places. Finally, if there are any organizations within your institute that provide career development, describe them since planning for your future career is a significant part of your training. Although this last resource is useful to graduate students, it is extremely important for inclusion as a resource for postdoctoral trainees, since part of their training will be the transition to their first independent academic position.

  - *Administrative support:* The support staff facilitates the day-to-day workings of a laboratory or a department. Most likely the business administrator assisted the applicant in putting together the budget and the final application. Departmental coordinators assist in organizing seminar series, reserving of rooms, etc. Briefly describe the administrative support staff available and how they will assist the applicant.

6.1.2 Equipment

As with the facilities, the reviewers need to see that you have all of the necessary equipment to perform the experiments described in your Research Training Plan. Very simply put, describe, in detail, the equipment at your disposal. Do not simply state "the laboratory has four PCR machines" but provide information on what make and model: "The laboratory has four Applied Biosystems Geneamp 9700 PCR machines." If you are using incubators for samples that require two different temperatures (e.g., bacteria vs. yeast) indicate that incubators maintained at these temperatures are present. If you are performing research that requires a specialized piece of equipment (e.g., immunofluorescent imaging), describe the microscope that will be used for this imaging and whether it is confocal or not. If there is equipment that belongs to the department, state "The following major equipment is present in the Department and will be available for the applicant's use." Of note, the level of detail indicated above is not necessary when describing standard items, such as refrigerators and freezers. However, with these items it is important to indicate that there are such storage areas available at a variety of different temperatures essential for storing different reagents and samples.

6.1.3 Institutional Environment and Commitment to Training (2 pages)

In addition to seeing that the technical and intellectual resources are available for the applicant, the reviewers need to see that the department and/or institute have a commitment to the applicant's success. Previously, an independent document that supplemented the information included in the Facilities, Equipment, and Sponsor/Cosponsor section was not necessary. However, the National Institutes of Health (NIH) now requires that an independent document be included in the application that describes the institutional, departmental, and laboratory environment along with a description of the educational programs for PhD and MD/PhD trainees (F30 and F31 applications). The inclusion of this separate document does not preclude including this information in the other places already described; however, this section does allow the applicant to expand on what is written elsewhere in the application to provide more detailed information.

Although much, if not all of the information included in this section is described in other parts of the application, this newly required section coalesces this information into one defined place, making it easier for a reviewer to evaluate the institutional environment. The NIH guidelines are very specific about what information is to be included here. It is necessary to discuss how the training will be undertaken within a laboratory with a well-established research program and a sponsor with a solid history of producing significant work in a field or topic that is related to the proposed project described in the Research Strategy. Information also needs to be included that describes opportunities for intellectual interactions with other laboratories and investigators. These interactions may include courses that will be taken, journal clubs, seminars, presentation requirements, and opportunities for attending seminars and meetings at regional institutions. It is also necessary to discuss the resources that are available for the applicant with respect to their research project, their career development, and for their educational advancement. As described above, although career development opportunities are important for graduate student applicants, they are essential for postdoctoral trainees.

For applicants submitting an F30 or F31application, this section must also include a subsection entitled "Educational Information." For PhD trainees (F31 and F31 diversity), this subsection needs to discuss the overall structure of the graduate program, including the number and nature of required courses, the milestones of the program (i.e., qualifying exams, preliminary exams, oral exams, committee meetings, etc.), the timeline of when these milestones occur, and any information detailing teaching that may be required of the applicant. It is also necessary to discuss the average time for students to complete their degree within each individual program and how the program will monitor the applicant's progress. Finally, describe the status of the applicant within this program. "The applicant is presently in the third year of the training program and as such has successfully passed her qualifying examination. She is on track to take her institutional preliminary exam in approximately 6 months time, at which point she will officially be a PhD candidate in the graduate program in Genetics."

For MD/PhD trainees (F30), this subsection needs to discuss the structure of the MD/PhD program at the institute. This information will include the years spent in clinical education, the manner in which the student will select a lab in which to perform their PhD research, the educational requirements during their PhD training (which may be very similar as described above for the F31 applications), and the subsequent timing and manner in which they transition back to the final years of medical education. As with many other sections in the grant application, it is important that MD/PhD trainees include explicit statements about the clinical aspects of their training environment. These aspects may include any clinical tutorials that they will take during the research years, any aspects of their research that will include clinical or translational content, the opportunities they will have to attend grand rounds, tumor boards, or any other clinical seminar or symposium, and most importantly, any activities or classes that are required by the MD/PhD program to assist them in transitioning back into the clinical years of their training once their research is completed.

Oftentimes institutes will already have a "boiler plate template" that may be used to assist in the writing of the Institutional Environment and Commitment to Training section. If one does not exist, it would beneficial for the program to develop such a document. Further, one of the most effective ways of constructing this section is to have the director of the graduate program, director of the MD/PhD program, the departmental graduate coordinator, or the department chair use the template provided by the institute (if one exists) or write this section for the applicant, including all of the information described above. Most importantly, even though a template may be used, *this information must be specialized for each individual trainee!* Obviously certain aspects of the program are the same for all trainees (i.e., classes, exams, milestones, etc.). However, the description of the research program and the trainee's progress through the program must be specific for that individual. Finally, the individual that provided this information must include their name, title, and role within the training program at the end of the document.

6.2 TRAINING POTENTIAL

Just as the Facilities and Resources, Equipment, and Institutional Environment and Commitment to Training is one of the most *objective* of criteria, the Training Potential is probably one of the most *subjective* of criteria during the review process. The Training Potential evaluates just that, the potential for the applicant to receive an exceptional training given the information provided in the entire grant application. In order to determine this potential, the reviewers consider all aspects of the training, including the applicant's qualities, the sponsor's qualifications, the sponsor's training plan, the institutional and intellectual environment, the technical aspects of the science, etc. The reason this section is the most subjective of the five major criteria is because of the natural bias and differences in opinion that exist in human nature and affect the review process (discussed in Chapter 2). As such, reviewers do not always view factors that contribute to the overall training potential with equal importance. Therefore, by some reviewers the Training Potential (along with the Institutional Environment) could be considered to carry a lower "weight" or influence on the overall strength of the application than the Applicant, Sponsor, and Research Training Plan. Alternatively, some reviewers may actually use the Training Potential to guide their decisions for the Overall Impact score.

Following are several examples of how the evaluation of the training potential of an application can differ depending on the personal biases and opinions of individual reviewers. Consider a situation where you have an exceptional predoctoral applicant (F31 grant); 4.0 undergraduate GPA, they published a first author paper from their undergraduate research, stellar letters of recommendation, mature career goals, and clear understanding of how the present training will help them achieve these goals. The Research Training Plan is top-notch, exceptionally written, highly significant, with well laid out experiments. However, despite the fact that the sponsor has been in his position for 9 years, he has only trained four students. Even though all four of the students have progressed to exceptional careers, this is considered by some reviewers to be a low to moderate training experience for the sponsor and will require the presence of a cosponsor. Therefore, despite the exceptional nature of the applicant and project, the perception of a "low training history" (or lack of sheer numbers of trainees) for the sponsor will negatively influence the training potential of the applicant for some reviewers.

Now, take as an example the situation where you have a postdoctoral applicant whose undergraduate grades weren't the greatest but improved throughout graduate school. Because of a difficult graduate project, the applicant took a little under 7 years to complete their degree and only published one first author paper. Despite letters of recommendation that attested to the fact that the graduate project was extremely difficult, thereby explaining the publication record, the longer graduate career and low publication record is seen as a deficit. The sponsor is a leader in the field, has trained over 20 postdoctoral fellows, and has a publication list of over 100 papers in highly respected journals. The Research Training Plan is considered to be one of the best seen in that study section. In this situation, some reviewers may consider the academic record of the applicant (regardless of the demonstrated improvement) and the numbers of publications (suggesting a "poor" productivity despite solid explanations to the contrary) to be highly important for determining how successful the applicant will be and how much they will be able to profit from the overall training plan.

Finally, you may have an applicant that is extremely strong, a sponsor who is a leader in their field and has trained large numbers of students to highly productive careers. However, the Research Training Plan is poorly written, lacks focus, has specific aims that are interdependent, and rely on experimental models that are in development and have not be proven to be feasible. Some reviewers may state that because of the strength of the sponsor and the applicant, the quality of the science may not be as critical to the overall training. However, many reviewers will look at the Research Training Plan and conclude that the quality of the scientific writing indicates that poor mentoring was involved in putting together the project and therefore, the training potential of this application is diminished.

These previous examples may be considered by some to be extreme; however, they are real life examples from study sections and have contributed to significantly lowered scores for the Training Potential. Of course more subtle concerns can come into play when a reviewer is considering the training potential of a grant. A training program at an institute may not include professional development and/or journal clubs causing the Institutional Environment to affect the Training Potential. The sponsor's training plan, even though it provides details, may not provide *enough* details or may be perceived to be "copied and pasted" from another grant, therefore not considered to be personal enough. Alternatively, the training plan may focus entirely on the technical aspects of the training and may not discuss other aspects of professional development. Any of these situations may result in lowering the score of the Training Potential. Of course, in all of these examples, the mindset of the reviewers as they are reading your grant will absolutely contribute to how strongly they feel each of these issues affect the training potential (discussed in Chapter 2). Alternatively, discussions in study section may bring to light issues that the reviewer may not have considered, also resulting in a lowered score.

6.3 OVERALL IMPACT SCORE

After evaluating each of the individual criteria described above and providing a score for each of these sections, the reviewers provide an Overall Impact Score. Like the determination of the score for the Training Potential, the Overall Impact Score takes into consideration all of the sections of the entire grant package: Applicant, Sponsor, Research Training Plan, Training Potential, and Institutional Environment. It must be noted that the overall impact score is NOT the average of the scores of the individual components. Instead, it is a score that each individual reviewer feels represents the true impact that the application will have on the overall training of the individual. Along these lines, many applicants are confused, and possibly even angry, when they receive their Summary Statement and find that the Overall Impact Score is actually lower than each of the individual scores. However, it is important to remember that ALL of the sections are taken into consideration and examined for how they will contribute to the overall training of the individual.

For example, consider the case where the applicant is excellent and received a score of a 3; the sponsor is solid but wrote a moderate training plan and receives a score of a 3; the Research Training Plan was average and had several weaknesses and also received a 3; the Institution is solid with no weaknesses and received a 1; and the Training Potential was considered to be a 3. However, the Overall Impact score was given a 4. Remember the scoring rubric presented in Chapter 2. While each of the individual components, by strict adherence to the rubric, are considered "very strong with some minor weaknesses" (score of a 3), when the application is considered as a whole, each section that individually contained *some minor weaknesses* translates into an overall application with *numerous minor weaknesses*. Again using strict adherence to the rubric, "strong with numerous minor weaknesses" equates to a score of a 4. As with the

Training Potential and as discussed in Chapter 2, the biases of the reviewers, the mindset of the reviewer while they are evaluating the application, and opinions of how strongly a reviewer feels different criteria will affect an overall impact come into play and cannot be predicted. Further, discussions in the study section (should the grant be discussed) will also alter the initial impact score provided by some reviewers to result in the final impact score presented to the applicant.

6.4 OTHER SCORED ITEMS

In addition to the five major criteria that receive individual scores, there are other items within the grant application that are considered scored items but do not individually receive a score. That is, these are items that may be considered when determining a score for the Research Training Plan, the Training Potential, or the Overall Impact score but do not carry as much weight as the five major criteria. These additional scored items include Vertebrate Animals and the Resource Sharing Plan.

6.4.1 Vertebrate Animals

If the Research Training Plan proposes the use of an animal model, then it is a requirement that your application includes a section that justifies the species being used, the numbers of animals required, veterinary care that will be provided, the procedures that will be used to ensure the minimization of pain and discomfort, the criterion to be used to implement euthanasia, and the method by which euthanasia will be performed. As with every other part of the grant application, this section requires the inclusion of details:

- *Proposed use of animals:* Provide detailed information describing how the animals will be used for the studies described in the Research Training Plan, including the species, strain, age, sex, and numbers of animals to be used in the proposed work. For example, if your Research Training Plan proposes the use of primary cells derived from neonate mice, you must provide a description of the strain of mice that will be used, the breeding process you will use to obtain the neonate mice, how many neonate pups are needed, the days post birth at which the mouse pups will be euthanized, how the pups will be euthanized to harvest the tissue, and the surgical procedures that you will use to obtain the tissue from which you will derive the primary cells. Further, if your studies require the use of only one sex (male vs. female), you must provide a rationale for why this selection is necessary.

• *Justification of the use of animal, species, and number of animals:* Provide detailed information describing why the proposed use of animal is required and a justification for the numbers of animals to be used in the study. Since animal work is costly and in many cases time-consuming, the reviewers, and the NIH, want to see a solid rationale for the use of animals and that similar studies could not be more effectively performed in a cellular model. Solid statements of rationale may be "The use of animal models is essential for understanding the complex process of differentiation. There is presently no in vitro system that can adequately model the disease state in a physiological environment. Further, this animal model has been chosen because the disease state induced in this model closely parallels the disease state observed in humans and therefore will provide highly relevant translational information." Alternatively, to continue the example used above, "Although alternatives to primary myoblasts exist in the form of cell lines, these lines are partially differentiated and have been manipulated and cultured to achieve immortality, resulting in the accumulation of genetic mutations that may alter the molecular characteristics of the transcription factor under investigation." In essence, you must demonstrate why there is no other alternative to the animal model system you propose to use. In addition, you must provide detailed information on the numbers of animals to be used within your study. This includes the number of animals required for the determination of statistical significance within sets, the total number of sets to be used (controls, mutants, various conditions, etc.), with a total animal count to comprise the entire study.

• *Veterinary care:* Provide information on the number of veterinarians on site, their availability in the case of an emergency, how frequently the animals will be inspected by either the veterinarian or a veterinary technician, and who these inspectors will report to should they observe any abnormalities (i.e., the attending veterinarian and/ or the principal investigator). This section must also include a description of how the animals will be housed (e.g., "All mice are housed in top filter ventilated cages on paper bedding with nestlets and breeding huts when necessary").

- *Procedures for limiting discomfort, pain, and distress:* If your proposed use of animals involves surgical procedures or procedures in which the animals will be restrained, you must provide a description of how the animals will be treated in order to minimize pain or discomfort. This includes describing the type of anesthetic that will be used for the surgery (i.e., general or local anesthesia, the amounts of anesthesia, and a rationale for why the type of anesthesia is being used) and how postsurgical pain will be managed and monitored. If animal restraint is required, a rationale for why restraint is unavoidable and a description of the method of restraint must be included. If you believe that the methods to be used will not generate pain or discomfort, this fact must be stated with a solid rationale for why this belief is the case.
- *Method of euthanasia:* If your studies involve a process that will generate a terminal condition (e.g., tumor formation), the endpoint of study itself involves extreme morbidity (e.g., extreme weight loss, weight gain, or muscle wasting), or each time point requires the sacrificing of the animal in order to harvest internal organs for analysis, then information describing the processes of euthanasia is required. This information must describe the drug and/or anesthetic that will be used, the amount of the drug, and whether the indicated level of drug is a lethal dose. Further, if extreme morbidity is expected, you must describe the parameters that will be used to determine that the animal must be euthanized to prevent further pain and suffering. These parameters may include, but are not limited to extreme weight loss (indicated by loss of a certain percentage of total body weight), unresponsiveness to immediate interventions, or extreme lethargy or inability to consume food or liquids. Finally, your description must explicitly state that the chosen method of euthanasia is consistent with the recommendations of the Panel on Euthanasia of the American Veterinary Medical Association.

6.4.2 Resource Sharing Plan

Many times the work performed in the Research Training Plan will generate unique resources, which can be in the form of reagents, such as antibodies or DNA constructs, model organisms, or large data sets, such as whole genome sequencing or genome-wide association studies.

The sharing of these unique resources is integral for the enhancement of research and facilitates advancing work in the field or science in general. When these unique resources have been developed through the use of NIH funds, it is a requirement that these resources be made readily available to the scientific community. The Resource Sharing Plan is the description of how you, the investigator, will make these reagents available to the scientific public. These methods of sharing may include placing the large data sets on a public access database for which a web address will be provided, sending of novel reagents when requested by an individual, or providing animals for breeding upon request.

CHAPTER 7

Details, Details, Details—Nonscored Items, Formatting, and the Cover Letter

Several components of the application package are considered "nonscored" items. These sections contain information that will be used by the National Institutes of Health (NIH) for public information purposes should your grant be funded (Project Summary and Project Narrative) or to ensure that your training will be in compliance with NIH guidelines (Responsible Conduct of Research). These items neither contribute to the individual scores nor will they influence the overall impact score of your grant application. However, it is still essential that the utmost care be used in writing each of these sections.

7.1 PROJECT SUMMARY/ABSTRACT (30 LINES)

The project summary is the abstract for the Research Training Plan and as such serves as a succinct description of the proposed work. Should the application be funded, the NIH will publish the Project Summary online on the NIH Reporter database (http://projectreporter.nih.gov/reporter.cfm). Therefore, the Project Summary must serve as a stand-alone document. Further, it must be written so that anyone scientifically or technically literate will be able to understand it. Because it serves as an overview of the project, the Project Summary must include background information, overall objectives, a statement of the hypothesis to be tested, the evidence or data that allowed the development of the hypothesis or supports the feasibility of the project, the Aims to be tested and the methods used to address these aims, and a reference to the health relatedness of the work.

Because the Project Summary succinctly summarizes the research project, it is often best to write this section after the Research Training Plan has been completed. Therefore, it is easy to take sentences written for the research plan and modify them slightly for the Project

A Practical Guide to Writing a Ruth L. Kirschstein NRSA Grant. DOI: https://doi.org/10.1016/B978-0-12-815336-9.00007-7

Summary. A general rubric that assists in constructing the Project Summary can be as follows:

- Begin the paragraph with two to three sentences describing the background of the project. You want to provide enough information so that the reader can understand the overall field and have perspective for how your project fits into this field. Along these lines, it is often good to lead off with a catchy sentence that highlights the severity of a disease or puts a scientific question in perspective as it relates to human health: "Chronic alcohol consumption alters metabolic regulation, which can lead to muscle wasting, one of the most recognized factors affecting morbidity in these individuals." To facilitate writing these opening sentences, it is helpful to condense and paraphrase the opening paragraph of your Specific Aims page.
- Once you have established the background, explicitly state the gap in knowledge and why this gap is a problem to advancing treatments: "However, the underlying molecular mechanisms that contribute to the development of chronic alcohol associated muscle wasting are not fully understood. Without this knowledge the ability to develop novel therapies to reduce morbidity associated with this condition will be greatly inhibited."
- Once you have stated the gap in knowledge, provide additional information from published literature evidence or preliminary data that allowed you to develop your hypothesis. This needs to be done in one to three sentences. As with the opening sentences, it is recommended to condense and paraphrase the literature evidence and preliminary data as stated on your Specific Aims page.
- Having provided the required information, state your hypothesis: "Therefore, we hypothesize that..." being very specific about what your hypothesis is. For example, if you are examining the role of a specific molecule in a signaling pathway and how that signaling is altered in a disease state: "Therefore, we hypothesize that the presence of chemokines in the proinflammatory environment associated with chronic alcohol consumption alters signaling ultimately disrupting the expression of genes associated with muscle wasting." It is recommended to use the exact wording for the statement of the hypothesis in the Project Summary that you used on the Specific Aims page.

- Then, state your specific aims: "We will address this hypothesis through the following Specific Aims…" making sure that the specific aims you describe here are written identically to those written in the Research Training Plan."
- Follow-up the statement of the aims with a very brief (one to two sentences) description of the experimental model system and how this model system will be used to address the aims. "We will utilize muscle satellite cells derived from our chronic binge alcohol animal model as our experimental model. We will treat these cells with proinflammatory cytokines and monitor molecules of the signaling pathway along with the transcriptional activity of the key transcription factor and the expression of genes essential for protein degradation."
- Wrap-up the paragraph by summarizing how you expect the successful completion of this project to advance the field and how this advancement will contribute to the health relevance of the disease and/or health-related issue you are studying. "The information obtained from this project will provide a solid groundwork to establish a model by which proinflammatory molecules contribute to muscle wasting. This model will thereby enable more detailed studies aimed at determining how these molecular mechanisms can be exploited to develop novel therapies to alleviate the morbidity associated with this disease."

After providing a statement of the health relevance of the project, applicants sometimes include a statement that describes how this project, or more generally the overall training plan, will provide a framework for an excellent training environment. This statement is not required and in fact the inclusion or failure to include such a statement does not detract from the overall summary.

7.2 PROJECT NARRATIVE (2–3 SENTENCES)

The Project Narrative is a statement that will be used for public dissemination and describes how your project is relevant to public health. This section is very short and consists of only two to three sentences. Because this element is used for public release, it must be written in a language that can be understood by the general, lay audience. Therefore, do not use jargon or highly technical terms but instead use broad language that focuses on the general impact that the project will have to a particular disease or health-related issues. For example: "Rhabdomyosarcoma is an aggressive childhood solid muscle tumor with a poor prognosis that is characterized by a specific oncogenic protein. Understanding how this oncogenic protein changes global miRNA and gene expression thereby altering transcriptional regulatory networks to affect normal muscle development will assist in identifying new targets that could be exploited for the rational design of drugs for the treatment of this tumor."

7.3 RESPONSIBLE CONDUCT OF RESEARCH (1 PAGE)

In 1989, the NIH established a policy concerning the teaching of responsible conduct of research. This policy requires that any training grant application must include a description of how the applicant will be instructed in the ethical issues related to basic research (http:// grants.nih.gov/grants/guide/notice-files/NOT-OD-10-019.html).   The responsible conduct of research encompasses many aspects of ethical behavior and is not limited to research misconduct, which refers to the fabrication, falsification, or plagiarism of work in proposals or published materials. Therefore, responsible conduct of research is the practice of scientific investigation with integrity and involves the awareness and application of established professional norms and ethical principles in the performance of ALL activities related to scientific research. Research training grants that lack a description of these types of instruction may be returned without review.

The NIH has established explicit information that is required for an acceptable description on the instruction in the Responsible Conduct of Research:

- **Class format:** Include a description of the format the instruction takes. Will the instruction include didactic lecture, group discussions, or both? What will be the source material for the lecture and/ or discussion (i.e., text book, essays, handouts)? How will performance in the class be determined (i.e., exam, take home essays, in class participation, etc.)?
- **Subject matter:** Include an explicit description of the topics to be covered in the instruction. This is most easily addressed by including a list of all of the lecture and/or class topics included in the courses the applicant will take, best found in the syllabus for the class. The

NIH does not have specific curricular requirements for the instruction. However, several topics are recommended that constitute satisfactory training. These topics include conflict of interest, use of human subjects or vertebrate animals, mentor/mentee responsibilities and relationships, collaborative research, peer review, laboratory tools and management, intellectual sharing and ownership, research misconduct, authorship on publications, and the scientist as a responsible member of society.

- *Faculty participation:* Include a description of how faculty will participate in the instruction. Will a single faculty member lead the class? Will several faculty members contribute in a team-taught format each lecturing on a topic given their area of expertise?
- *Duration of instruction:* Provide a description of how long the class and/or instruction will last (i.e., 6 weeks, one semester, etc.)
- *Frequency of instruction:* Provide a description of how frequently the class will meet. This information can be combined with the duration as in the following example: "The course met/will meet for 1 h each week for the duration of the fall semester."

In addition to the formal instruction just described, it is also acceptable to include a statement that is tailored to the individual applicant and includes one-on-one mentoring from the sponsor as it relates to general scientific integrity or ethical issues associated with the specific research activities. While these latter discussions are acceptable as supplementary information, one-on-one instruction with the mentor *will not* be considered a substitute for formal classroom instruction. Further, as the Responsible Conduct of Research is not a scored item, a poorly written section will not prevent the funding of an otherwise exceptional grant. The applicant will simply have to rectify the problematic issues to be acceptable to the NIH before the grant is officially awarded.

7.4 FORMATTING

The NIH has very specific guidelines regarding formatting and these guidelines apply to all sections of the grant application. These guidelines are in place to make sure consistency exists in the presentation of grant applications, thereby facilitating the ease with which the applications can be read. These guidelines also prevent the utilization of smaller fonts that would allow increased amounts of information to be included within the application, thereby providing equity between all grant applications. These formats are to be strictly adhered to and failure to do so may result in the grant being administratively rejected without review. These formatting specifications are as follows:

- *Font:* Arial, Helvetica, Palatino Linotype, or Georgia typeface, 11 point or larger, with a black font color.
- *Type density:* May be no more than six lines per inch, which equates roughly to a single spaced distance between lines of type.
- *Paper size and margins:* 8.5″ × 11″ paper size is required with a minimum of 0.5-inch margins on top, bottom, left, and right.
- *Page formatting:* Use only a "single column" format (instead of double column format) and do not include headers or footers.
- *Page numbering:* It is not required. Page numbers will be system-generated in the complete application upon submission, with pages numbered sequentially for all parts of the grant.
- *Figures, Graphs, and Tables:* Figure legends, table descriptors, and text within graphs and charts may be smaller than the 11 point required for the body of the text. However, you must use the same font in the legends and descriptors as you do in the body of the text. Further, the font size cannot be any smaller than is legible when viewed at normal size or printed out onto 8.5″ × 11″ paper.
- *Page limits:* The page limits for each section, as dictated by the application guide are strictly adhered to. Failure to stay within these page limits will result in an administrative rejection without review.

In addition to these official formatting guidelines, it is important to keep in mind the overall appearance of the application. This fact was discussed previously in the presentation of figures in the Preliminary Data section of the Research Training Plan (see Chapter 5). However, this attention to overall appearance also comes into play in the actual text of the application, in particular in the visual density of the text and the complexity of writing. When constructing your application it is essential that you use shorter, more declarative statements that flow from one sentence and paragraph to the next and that you create "white space" in your text, thereby providing visual rest for the reader's eye.

To illustrate this point it's often good to keep in mind that you want to write like Hemingway, not Faulkner. Ernest Hemingway and William Faulkner, two giants of American literature, both Nobel laureates and Pulitzer Prize winners... two VERY different writing styles. William Faulkner revolutionized the way the English language was used in order to capture the workings of the human mind, many times describing a tortured mind in its descent into insanity using stream of consciousness writing. Hemingway examined how human kind react to harsh situations, how they exhibit "grace under pressure." Although both men captured the deep emotional, political, and social complexities of their time and world, they used very different writing styles in order to do this. Faulkner wrote long, complex, seemingly wandering sentences that covered several pages. These sentences were punctuated with parenthetical phrases, italics, and even a lack of punctuation to represent confusion and seemingly chaotic wanderings of the human mind. In contrast, Hemingway created and perfected what is now known as "shotgun prose." He used short declarative sentences that are straight to the point. However, these short declarative sentences flow to create a work that suggest deeper meanings than what is physically stated on the page. Hemingway said more through what was left unsaid, through the underlying meaning of the words on the page, than many authors are capable of doing in several pages of text.

Visually these writing styles are very different, too. Faulkner's writing appears very dense on the page, with paragraphs that go on for several pages leaving very little white space, or visual rest for the reader's eye. Hemingway's writing, on the other hand, has shorter paragraphs punctuated with dialog, thereby creating large amounts of white space and visual rest for the eye. It is this latter appearance that you need to strive for in the writing of your application. This can be done relatively easily:

- Provide a line of space between paragraphs.
- Write shorter paragraphs that contain one defined concept or idea and if you find that a paragraph consumes a majority of the page, find a way to break it up into smaller, bite sized thoughts and paragraphs.
- Use shorter, declarative sentences that flow one into the other, going for the "shot gun prose" style of Hemingway over the long, convoluted style of Faulkner. As with the paragraphs, if you find a sentence continuing on for many lines of text, find a way to grammatically separate it into individual sentences.

Although the concept of visual "white space" may not seem important, examine the difference in appearance between a Research Training Plan that does not follow this suggestion (Fig. 7.1) and one that does (Fig. 7.2). Remember, the person reviewing your grant may be approaching this task under adverse conditions. Opening an application and being faced with a dense page of text with little to no "breathing room" for the eye may seem very daunting to that reviewer, thereby giving them an unintentional negative first impression.

Figure 7.1 Illustration of minimal "white space" in a grant application.

will individually clone the IGF2, IGF-1R, St8sia2, NCAM, or Plxna2 promoters into a promoter-less luciferase reporter vector (pGL3-Basic). We will perform transcriptional assays by transiently transfecting each individual reporter construct into the RH30 ARMS tumor cell lines stably transduced with empty vector, wild-type Pax3-FOXO1, or the Pax3-SGXG46S201A or S201D). We will determine the extent of transcriptional activity by luciferase analysis as previously described by us[4,6]. To determine the ability of Pax3-FOXO1 or its phospho-mutants to bind to the promoter elements, we will perform a ChIP analysis on the described RH30 ARMS tumor cells. We will immunoprecipitate ectopic FLAG-Pax3-FOXO1 or its mutants with a FLAG-specific antibody and we will determine the presence of each individual promoter by PCR amplification of the immunoprecipitated complexes with primers specific for each of the promoters.

Experiment 3. Examine the mechanism by which IGF2/IGF-1R contributes to ARMS tumor phenotypes. To determine the contributions that IGF2 and IGF-1R make to in vitro ARMS cell migration, invasion, and anchorage independent growth, we will individually knockdown the expression of IGF2 or IGF-1R with commercially available shRNA specific to each gene (GeneCopoeia, Rockville, MD) in RH30 ARMS tumor cells. We will confirm efficient knockdown by qRT-PCR and Western blot analysis. We will also treat the cells with neutralizing antibodies specific for IGF2 (R & D Systems) or IGF-1R (Calbiochem), as previously described[17]. We will then determine the effect each of these treatments has on ARMS tumor cell migration, invasion, and anchorage independent growth, as described in the Preliminary Studies.

Experiment 4. Examine the mechanism by which St8sia2/NCAM contributes to ARMS tumor phenotypes. To determine the mechanism by which St8sia2 and NCAM contribute to ARMS tumor migration, invasion, and anchorage independent growth, we will individually knockdown the expression of St8sia2 or NCAM with commercially available shRNA (GeneCopoeia) in RH30 ARMS tumor cells and confirm knockdown of each as described above. We will also treat the cells with endoneuraminidase-N, an endosialidase that specifically degrades linear polymers of sialic acid via α-2,8-linkage associated with NCAM[13]. We will then determine the effect each of these treatments has on ARMS tumor cell migration, invasion, and anchorage independent growth, as described in the Preliminary Studies.

Experiment 5. Examine the mechanism by which Plxna2 contributes to ARMS tumor phenotypes. To determine the mechanism by which Plxn2 contributes to ARMS tumor migration, invasion, and anchorage independent growth, we will knockdown the expression of Plxna2 with commercially available shRNA (OriGene, Rockville, MD) in RH30 ARMS tumor cells and confirm knockdown of each as described above. To determine if Plxna2 mediates its effects through its interaction with the membrane bound Semaphorin 6A or as a co-receptor with neuropilin to interact with the secreted Semaphorin 3A we will knockdown the expression of Semaphorin 6A or neuropilin using shRNA specific to each gene (GeneCopoeia) or we will inhibit the interaction between Semaphorin 6A or Semaphorin 3A and Plxna2 using neutralizing antibodies against the individual Semaphorins, as previously described[8,9]. We will then determine the effect each of these treatments has on ARMS tumor cell migration, invasion, and anchorage independent growth.

Expected Outcomes: Based on our differential gene analysis (Preliminary Studies) and previous literature evidence we expect to observe a decrease in expression of IGF2, IGF-1R, St8sia2, NCAM, and Plxna2 upon shRNA knockdown of Pax3-FOXO1 in the ARMS tumor cell lines. We also expect to observe an increase in expression of these genes upon the ectopic expression of Pax3-FOXO1 in the ERMS tumor cell line. Further, based on our observation that the inhibition of phosphorylation of Pax3-FOXO1 at Ser201 suppresses tumor cell migration, invasion, and anchorage independent growth, and given the known biological functions of these genes, we expect to observe a decrease in expression of these five genes in ARMS cells ectopically expressing Pax3-FOXO1(S201A) relative to wild-type Pax3-FOXO1. Consistent with this expectation, we predict that Pax3-FOXO1(S201A) will have a decreased ability to activate expression of the gene promoters, as determined by luciferase and ChIP analysis. Finally, we expect that the specific knockdown of each inhibitory gene along with the described inhibitory treatments, will suppress ARMS tumor cell migration, invasion, and anchorage independent growth, as illustrated in our Preliminary Studies.

Potential Problems and Alternative Strategies: Literature evidence and our Preliminary Studies support the idea that IGF2, IGF-1R, St8sia2, NCAM, and Plxna2 are regulated in a Pax3-FOXO1-dependent manner and contribute to in vitro ARMS migration, invasion, and anchorage independent growth. Along these lines, a

Figure 7.2 Illustration of the inclusion of "white space" in a grant application.

In contrast, the visible white space on the page immediately lets them feel that they can read and digest your writing in small, discrete sections, which can be a relief for a tired reviewer.

One last thing to consider when writing your application—be very sparing with the use of acronyms! While acronyms can be good when writing a document with very limited space constraints, the use of too many acronyms can become overly confusing, ultimately annoying what may be a very tired reviewer. Remember, although the acronyms that you use may be familiar to you and to people in your field, these same acronyms will not necessarily be familiar to the person reading your application, who most likely is not in your field. When you use acronyms you are asking the reader to remember their meaning as they read through the application. The use of too many acronyms therefore can become burdensome on the reader, many times requiring them to search back through the document to remind themselves of their original definition. Therefore, a good rule of thumb is if you know that a term will be used continually throughout the document [e.g., fluorescence in situ hybridization (FISH)] then use the acronym, spelling it out the first time it is encountered with the acronym immediately following it in parentheses. If you know that the term will be used minimally (e.g., only once or twice), then it is better to simply spell out the term.

7.5 COVER LETTER

Part of ensuring that the grant application receives a fair review is making sure that it is sent to the most appropriate study section. As described in Chapter 2, a majority of the study sections associated with the Ruth L. Kirschstein training grants are interdisciplinary and therefore focus on a particular scientific topic and/or discipline. While some of these disciplines may overlap, they each have a very distinct focus. As such, the reviewers on these panels have very different ways of thinking about science. For example, a grant may contain a research training plan that discusses the role of a transcription factor in regulating gene expression during muscle development. The research examines a molecular mechanism important in muscle development and proposes experiments that are molecular biological and biochemical in nature. Technically, this grant should be directed to the study section on Genes, Genomes, and Genetics, which review grants that relate to the regulation of gene expression. However, because the research examines transcriptional regulation in the context of muscle development, it could also be considered for the study section on Cell Biology and Development.

On the surface either section would seem appropriate. However, consider the research focus of the members of these study sections. Many reviewers on the Genes, Genomes, and Genetics study section perform molecular biological, biochemical, and genetic work and can therefore appreciate the line of proposed experiments. In contrast, many of the members on the Cell Biology and Development study section perform more developmental biology work and would expect and/or want to see a line of experiments that utilize more developmental biology. Although it seems as if assignment to the latter section would be okay, in actuality, the grant may not receive an appropriate review simply due to differences in scientific experience.

The assignment of grant applications to study sections occurs in the Division of Receipt and Referral at the Center for Scientific Review. It is within this division that the content of the scientific plan is examined and a decision as to the most appropriate study section is made. Since people who are not intimately familiar with the work are making decisions on where the application is assigned, the applicant can facilitate this process, and influence the assignment of the application, by requesting a study section and providing explicit logic within the cover letter as to why this section is the most appropriate. Along these lines, the NIH has developed a recommended format when including assignment requests in the cover letter, which is as follows:

"Please accept for consideration the Ruth L. Kirschstein National Research Service Awards for Individual Predoctoral Fellows (Parent F31) grant application entitled [insert title] in response to announcement [insert the NIH program announcement number].

> *Please assign this application to the following:*
> *Institute/Center:*
> > *National Cancer Institute—NCI*
> *Scientific Review Group:*
> > *IMST—Interdisciplinary Molecular Sciences and Training Fellowship: Oncological Sciences [F09]*
> *The reasons for this request are. ..."*

Follow this statement by one short paragraph outlining your rationale for this request. When describing the rationale, it is often advisable to quote directly from the description of the topics covered by that study section. "The stated focus of the Oncological Sciences IMST study section is to 'review applications involving the pathology of the malignant cell... with an emphasis on mechanisms... and molecular events in gene regulation.' Among the stated specific areas covered are 'gene regulation including... transcription... relevant to oncogenesis.'" This rationalization is followed by a second short paragraph in which you briefly describe the research in the proposal and state exactly how this research fits within the scope of the topics considered by the desired study section. Finally, a cover letter for the Ruth L. Kirschstein training grants also requires the inclusion of the name, degree, position, and affiliation of the individuals who have agreed to submit reference letters.

CHAPTER 8

Now What?—Resubmission

Once you've submitted your grant, then the waiting begins. Grants submitted for the April 8 deadline will be assigned to a study section approximately a month later. Once assigned, these study sections will meet anywhere between late June and mid-July. The study section will last 1−2 days, depending on the number of grants under consideration, after which the Scientific Review Officer must compile the scores for notification. Once compiled, these scores will be posted on individual eRA Commons sites, a process which may take another week or longer. However, at this point the applicant will only know whether their grant was "not discussed," whether they received a score and if so, what that score is. Further, unless the score is better than 20, the applicant will also not know with absolute certainty whether the grant will be funded. As discussed in Chapter 2, each individual institute determines the funding levels and what scores will be funded. In addition, the applicant will not know why they received the score they did as the reviews, in the form of a Summary Statement, will not be released for about another month. Therefore, it may be upwards of 3.5−4 months from the time a grant application is submitted until receipt of the critiques.

Before discussing the Summary Statement and how to address comments, a brief discussion of how the final score is presented is needed. As described up to this point, the reviewers provide single integer numbers from 1 to 9 for each of the individual components and for the overall impact score. These single integer numbers are used in study section to establish a range for voting. When the final votes are entered following discussion, each member submits their decision as a single digit number from 1 to 9. As described in Chapter 2, the entries from all of the members are then averaged to provide the final score for a particular grant. When reported to the applicant, the score is multiplied by 10. For example, assume there are eight members on a study

A Practical Guide to Writing a Ruth L. Kirschstein NRSA Grant. DOI: https://doi.org/10.1016/B978-0-12-815336-9.00008-9

section. After discussion the scores these members enter are 1, 2, 4, 3, 3, 2, 2, and 3. This range of scores would result in an average score of 2.5, which would then be reported to the applicant as a score of 25.

8.1 THE SUMMARY STATEMENT

The Summary Statement is the document that summarizes the overall review of the applicant's grant. If the application received a score, which means that the proposal was discussed in the study section, the statement will begin with a paragraph entitled "Resume and Summary of Discussion." This paragraph is written by the Scientific Review Officer and summarizes the discussion that occurred for this grant during the meeting, detailing the score driving factors with respect to strengths and weakness of the grant application. If the grant did not receive a score, which means that it was not discussed, there will be no summary included.

Following the summary of the discussion, the Summary Statement next presents the critiques of each of the three reviewers who read your application. These reviews are separated into Reviewer #1, Reviewer #2, and Reviewer #3 with each section beginning with a listing of the five different criteria (Fellowship Applicant, Sponsors/Collaborators/Consultants, Research Training Plan, Training Potential, Institutional Environment and Commitment to Training) and the individual priority score (1–9) that the reviewer assigned to each individual criterion. This score description is followed by a paragraph entitled "Overall Impact/Merit" in which the reviewer summarizes their opinion of the overall quality of the application with statements of what they felt the strengths of the application were and what weaknesses detracted from the overall quality of the grant. Next in the Summary Statement are individual sections with headings for each of the five criteria. Under these headings are subheadings for "Strengths" and "Weaknesses," where the reviewer provides bulleted, detailed, and hopefully constructive comments about what they felt were the strengths and/or weaknesses for that particular section in the application. Completing the Summary Statement will be a list of the members of the study section with their academic rank and affiliation. Remember, these reviews are anonymous, which means that although you know who was on the study section, you will not know which members of the study section reviewed your application.

As discussed in Chapter 2, only Reviewers #1 and #2 are required to provide individual scores for each criterion, provide an overall impact statement, and fully comment on the strengths and weaknesses of each of the individual sections. Reviewer #3 needs only to provide individual scores and write an overall impact statement. In a perfect world, all of the reviewers would provide solid, rational, detailed, and constructive comments that will direct the applicant in addressing the perceived weaknesses of the grant. Further, the comments provided should also justify and/or coincide with the scores given based on the NIH scoring rubric. However, the reality is that many times an applicant will receive reviews for a section in which "no weaknesses were noted." The absence of any noted weakness, if strict adherence to the NIH rubric was followed, should coincide with a score of a 1. However, many times even though a reviewer noted no weaknesses, they will still give a score of a 3 for that section. A score of a 3 indicates that minor weaknesses should be present and require a rationalization for why that score was given.

It is also possible that even though the comments and scores coincide as described in the scoring rubric, the comments are vague or indicate that the reviewer has not carefully read the application. For example, a grant could be submitted in which the sites of protein modification have been identified and published. Based on this published knowledge, the Research Training Plan then focuses on determining the biological relevance of each of these identified protein modifications. In the review the application receives a comment, "The proposal could focus more on the overall importance of the modification rather than just identifying specific sites of modification." It is apparent that the reviewer did not read the application closely or if they did, they were not careful in writing a proper critique. These types of inconsistencies are frustrating and ultimately not necessarily fair. However, fair or not, the discussion of human nature and natural biases that occur during the review process must be kept in mind and ultimately it is the job of the applicant to address the concerns of these reviews.

8.2 TO RESUBMIT OR NOT TO RESUBMIT

The question to resubmit is always important to ask when receiving the results and reviews of a grant application. Sometimes the question is very easy to answer. If the grant received a score of 20 or better it will most likely be funded and resubmission is not necessary. Conversely, if a grant is not discussed and the reviewers consistently gave individual scores of 5 or worse, a resubmission of the grant would most likely be a futile exercise. However, there are definitely gray areas where the decision to resubmit may not be as cut and dried as the two scenarios just given. As with all aspects of submitting a Ruth L. Kirschstein training grant, the decision to resubmit is a case-by-case basis and will be different for each application depending on the comments and critiques.

When deciding whether to resubmit, it is important to remember how the decision to discuss grants is determined (see Chapter 2). If there are <8−10 applications for a particular section (i.e., F30, F31, F32, etc.), all of the grants will be discussed and as such all of the grants within this section will receive a score. Therefore, a grant may receive a score, but that score may be a 60 or worse. In this case, it would not necessarily be beneficial to resubmit since overall that application was perceived as being significantly flawed. In contrast, if there are more than 8−10 grants (as with the F32 postdoctoral grants which may have upward of 60−70 submissions in a study section), then only the top ≈ 50% of the grants will be discussed with the cutoff point being determined by how the scores naturally divide. In this situation, it is highly possible that a grant may not be discussed but in actuality have received an initial impact score in the low 30s, which technically may be close to a fundable level as some institutes within the NIH may fund grants that have scores in the upper 20s. In this latter illustration, this application would definitely be worth revising for resubmission.

The next question that arises is if the application was not discussed, in which case the initial impact score cannot be known, how does one determine if the overall impression of the study section was favorable and that the grant is worth resubmitting? An examination of the individual criterion scores from each reviewer will indicate the overall impression. Further, chances are that a majority of the reviewers' comments will be constructive and detailed, providing insight into the strengths and weaknesses of the grant. Therefore, if a majority of the individual criterion scores are 4s, 3s, or 2s with solid, positive critiques and these critiques are easily addressable in a revision, then the overall impression was favorable and resubmission should be considered. Even if a not-discussed grant has poor individual criterion scores and unfavorable critiques, it is possible that a grant application could be rewritten and revised significantly to improve its score. Ultimately, the decision to resubmit is up to each individual applicant and sponsor and needs to be determined based on the general impressions given through the Summary Statement.

8.3 ADDRESSING THE CRITIQUES

During the review process, a resubmitted grant will be given an A1 status (i.e., CA123456-A1), which indicates that the application in front of the reviewer is a resubmission. As a resubmission, there is one additional criterion added to the review process, a criterion that does not receive its own individual score but whose evaluation contributes to the overall impact score: How well did the resubmitted application address the previous reviewers' comments? When a reviewer is evaluating a resubmitted grant, they will have access to the Summary Statement from the previous submission, which will allow them to know the previous reviewers opinions of the strengths and weaknesses of the previous submission. Whether these prior critiques were addressed or the quality with which these previous critiques were addressed will then be considered in the resubmitted form.

At this point, an important note must be made about the reviewing of resubmitted grants. The makeup of study sections for the Ruth L. Kirschstein grants is ad hoc, which means that the composition is not constant and usually changes from study section to study section. There will be several members who routinely serve on a particular study section; however, none of the members is assigned to a single section on a permanent basis. Therefore, it is more than likely that the people who reviewed a grant application on the first submission will NOT review the grant upon resubmission. Further, even among the reviewers who have served on multiple study sections for the same topic, it is highly unlikely that they will be assigned a resubmitted grant on which they served as one of the original reviewers. Finally, even if a person is assigned a resubmitted grant that they reviewed on its first submission, they will not necessarily remember having reviewed it the first time around. Remember, it has been approximately 4 months or longer since they would have originally seen this grant. If they were not able to serve on the subsequent study section, upwards of 8 months may have elapsed. In that time period, they will have reviewed at least 24 (or more) other grants and discussed about 100 grants (or more) in total. It is a good rule of thumb when rewriting a grant for resubmission, in particular in writing the Introduction (see below), to assume that the person reading the resubmission will not have seen the original submission and if they did, they will not remember having seen it before. Therefore, the assessment of the resubmission, regardless of who is reading it, will rely almost solely on the previous critiques and how well these critiques were addressed.

In the world of sales, there is a saying that the customer is always right. When an applicant sits down to revise a grant for resubmission a similar saying could apply: The reviewer is always correct. In essence, if the reviewer says jump, the applicant should say "how high." These sayings are not meant to be taken literally. Of course there are situations in which a reviewer will provide a critique that makes it evident that they did not fully understand the point that was being made or simply did not read the grant carefully enough. However, the saying above is meant to indicate that if the reviewer wrote a critique, regardless of how much you agree or disagree with it, this critique must be taken into consideration when revising the grant and must be addressed in the revision. If not, neglecting to do so will be noted when the resubmission goes to study section and this neglect may negatively influence the overall score.

When revising a proposal, it is very important that the applicant tries their best to put their pride away and approach the process with the perspective that the reviewer's comments are valid and are intended to improve the grant. Sometimes this mind set needs to develop over a short period of time after the initial shock, anger, and frustration of the score and the perceived injustice of the comments wears off. However, even in the case where a comment is made by a reviewer that suggests careless reading, the applicant would do well to take a step back, dissociate themselves from what was written in the first submission, and make the assumption that they did not present their point as clearly or logically as they thought they did. In essence, the reviewer was correct, maybe not in what they said or how they said it, but in the sense that they highlighted something that needs to be improved for clarity.

Some of the critiques are straightforward to address. If a sponsor has a moderate but not stellar training history and a reviewer comments on this fact, then in the resubmission, a cosponsor needs to be included using all of the qualifications discussed in Chapter 4. If the sponsor does not have funding to cover the entirety of the training period, they must include solid and detailed descriptions for exactly how the applicant will be supported financially. If there are experimental issues that were called into question, the Research Training Plan must be modified according to the critiques. If the applicant proposes the use of a cutting-edge technique but provides no evidence that the expertise is present in the lab or at the institute to perform the experiments or to evaluate the results, then a collaborator must be included in the resubmission along with a letter of support. If it is felt that there is not enough preliminary data to support the feasibility of the project, this preliminary data must be included in the resubmission. It is through these critiques that the reviewers are telling the applicant exactly what is needed to improve the application.

There are other situations that may not necessarily be as easy to address. If a reviewer comments about the poor academic performance of the applicant, there is nothing that can be done to change this fact (see Chapter 3). The past is the past. However, the applicant can address this issue by providing a statement in the revised Personal Statement about why they had a poor academic history and how this history will not or does not affect their present and future capabilities as an independent scientist. The applicant could also have a referee from his previous institute comment that the previous academic performance is not reflective of their current ability. In another case, an applicant has chosen to remain at their graduate institute to perform their postdoctoral work, a situation that is not looked upon favorably by reviewers. Therefore, in the revision include a statement in the Personal Statement of the Biosketch and the Selection of Sponsor and Institute as to why this choice was made and provide evidence that the present training is different from past training experiences (e.g., different department, different model system, etc.). Regardless of the critique, the issue that the critique raised must be addressed and it must be addressed in a logical, clear, and very prominent manner.

Finally, sometimes the reviewer is just wrong or sometimes there are simply just differences in opinion or differences in the interpretation of data or experimental design between the applicant and the reviewer. Although the first instinct is to merely brush aside the critique as being unfounded or wrong and ignore it, the comment must be addressed. However, because these are differences in opinion or cases where the reviewer simply did not take note of something that was already in the grant, these issues need not be addressed directly in the body of the application. Instead, they should be professionally and respectfully addressed in the section called "Introduction to the Application" (see below). Ultimately, if the reviewer has commented on any aspect of the application, that comment must be considered and addressed in some form or another within the revised application.

8.4 INTRODUCTION TO THE APPLICATION (1 PAGE)

A resubmitted grant is required to have an additional section entitled "Introduction to the Application." It is within this section that the applicant specifically details how they have addressed the critiques of the reviewers from the original submission. This section is extremely important because, as described above, it is very possible that the reviewers reading the resubmitted application most likely were not the people who read the original submission and if they were, they will not necessarily remember the details. Therefore, it is critical that the Introduction be carefully written to concisely point out the deficiencies noted in the first submission, explicitly point out how these deficiencies were addressed, and direct the reader to the place in the revised application where the modifications were incorporated.

When writing the Introduction, it is good to start with a sentence reminding the reviewer that they are, in fact, reading a resubmission and when the previous submission occurred: "This is a revised version of the proposal [enter the assigned grant number], which was originally submitted in August of 20XX." This information provides the reader with a time frame between the original submission and the present resubmission, which allows them to evaluate whether the amount of productivity seen in the revision is consistent with the time that the applicant had to produce the work. Follow this statement by briefly pointing out the strengths of the original submission by using exact quotes from the previous reviewers: "Several strengths were noted, in particular that the original submission was 'focused and significant,' as well as 'an excellent proposal from an excellent applicant working in an excellent environment under the sponsorship of an excellent, well-funded mentor.'"

Once the strengths of the original submission are noted, be sure to respectfully recognize the value of the critiques of the previous reviewers: "In addition to these strengths several criticisms were presented, which we have addressed and subsequently produced what we feel to be an improved proposal." At this point provide either a bulleted or numbered list of the previous critiques with a concise, yet detailed description of how these critiques have been addressed. It is a good idea to explicitly quote the previous reviews, or an abbreviated form of the previous reviews, to provide evidence of what was said and include detailed information regarding where in the resubmission the reader will find these modifications:

> *"**Reviewer #1**: The biological significance of the proposed mutations is not clear beyond the information already known.*
> **Response**: We provide solid experimental data demonstrating the biological significance of the mutations at each individual site as it relates to the known biological properties of the cellular model (Table 3.1 and Figures 2 and 4)."

When addressing the critiques there are three general types of responses that are needed depending on the nature of the critique: (1) addressing critiques that explicitly change and/or modify the original proposal; (2) addressing critiques that cannot be changed; and (3) addressing critiques in which there is an honest difference in opinion between the applicant and the reviewer. Each of these situations needs to be handled differently when writing the Introduction. The first situation, in which there is the inclusion of additional data to support the point, or the addition of a cosponsor to augment what was considered a poor training history, are fairly straightforward, as illustrated in the above example. The second situation is probably the most difficult to address since this usually involves problems with the history of the applicant that can no longer be changed. In this case, it is best to directly recognize the point that was made by the reviewer and then provide information that will dispel their concerns: "I recognize that my grades in my undergraduate years were not optimal. However, during this time I was dealing with several personal issues that distracted my focus (see applicant Personal Statement). Once these personal issues were resolved, and my focus returned, my academic performance improved, as evidenced by my improved grades in graduate school." This statement recognizes that a problem existed, it provides an explanation that any human being would understand, and it demonstrates that this apparent setback was temporary and does not affect the present training period or the future prospects of the applicant.

The third situation, while apparently straightforward to address, is also the trickiest. In the situation where there are differences in scientific opinion between the reviewer and the applicant, no direct modifications are necessarily made to the application. Therefore, the viewpoint or opinion of the applicant needs to be explicitly stated in the Introduction where the applicant is arguing their opinion to the new reviewer. Ultimately, the new reviewer makes the decision on who they think is correct, a decision that is based on the previous critiques, the applicant's rebuttal, and their own interpretation from reading the application. However, it is still possible to write the response such that the scientific point is made respectfully and ultimately assuming the viewpoint that the original logic may not have been written as clearly as it could have been. "The applicant respectfully disagrees with this reviewer's assessment of the data. In the original application we stated that [explicitly quote the statement from the original submission]. Along these lines, we feel that literature evidence firmly supports the conclusion that [state the conclusion that you believe to be correct]. However, the interpretation of the results may have resulted from a lack of clarity in the writing. Therefore, we have revised the writing for clarity and included additional references to support our conclusion."

Of course these three scenarios are generalizations. However, a majority of the critiques will usually fall under these three broad concepts. As with all sections of the application, the type of responses that are required will be different for each individual application and applicant and may not necessarily be easy to address. Regardless of how much the applicant agrees with the critiques or feels that the critiques are fair, it is essential to address the reviewers' comments head on rather than ignore any of them. The reviewers of the resubmission usually read the applications very carefully, especially a revised application, and very little will get past them. The neglect of a previous comment by the applicant will be noted and most times will negatively affect the review of the resubmission. In fact the scores for a majority of resubmitted grants do not improve significantly, or even are poorer relative to the original submission simply because the applicant did not feel it was necessary to address all of the critiques.

Another note that must be made is that many times the nature of the three reviewers' comments is very similar. For example, all three may comment on poor grades or lack of publications. Two of the three may have commented on the quality of a particular experiment or the funding status of the sponsor. If this is the case, it is recommended that instead of discussing the critiques by individual reviewers that you group your comments in the Introduction by topic. For example: "It was noted by two of the reviewers that the applicant's grades were less than optimal during the first two undergraduate years. I have addressed this concern by stating that I experienced personal issues during that time period of my education and I have addressed it more in depth in the Personal Statement of my Biosketch." Remember, you only have one page to describe how you addressed all of the reviewers' comments and it is essential that you condense wherever possible without sacrificing clarity and detail.

Finally, it is essential that you conclude the Introduction by informing the reader how you are indicating changes within the grant: "All modifications to the grant are indicated by a solid black line in the left hand margin." Include the indicated markings wherever you have modified the grant. It is usually not recommended to utilize bold, underlined, or italicized font to indicate where the modifications occur. As discussed before, these types of modified fonts are used to provide stress and bring attention to key points and statements that you are making (e.g., hypothesis or significance). Further, a large amount of bolded, italicized, or underlined sections may look messy and overly busy.

CHECKLIST OF REQUIRED ITEMS

The following is a checklist of the major application components required for all Ruth L. Kirschstein Training grants (F30, F31, F31 Diversity, and F32) that must be written by either the applicant or the sponsor.

APPLICANT'S RESPONSIBILITY

- Research Training Plan
  - Introduction (resubmissions only—1 page)
  - Specific Aims (1 page)
  - Research Strategy (6 pages)
    - Significance
    - Approach
  - Human Subjects (only if human studies proposed)
  - Vertebrate Animals (only if animal studies proposed)
  - Bibliography and References Cited (no page limitations)
- Resource Sharing Plan (1 page)
- Facilities (1 page)
- Equipment (1 page)
- Institutional Environment and Commitment to Training (2 pages)
- Respective Contributions (1 page)
- Applicant's Background and Goals for Fellowship Training (6 pages)
  - Doctoral Dissertation and Research Experience
  - Training Goals and Objectives
  - Activities Planned Under This Award
- Selection of Sponsor and Institute (1 page)
- Responsible Conduct of Research (1 page)
- Cover Letter (1 page)
- List of Referees (3 referees minimum)
- Applicant's Biosketch (5 pages)

- Descriptive Title (200 characters in length, including spaces and punctuation)
- Project Summary/Abstract (30 lines of text)
- Project Narrative (2–3 sentences in layman's terms)

SPONSOR/COSPONSOR RESPONSIBILITY

- Sponsor and Cosponsor Information (6 pages)
  - Research Support Available
  - Sponsor's/Cosponsor's Previous Fellows/Trainees
  - Training Plan, Environment, Research Facilities
  - Number of Fellows/Trainees During the Fellowship
  - Applicant's Qualifications and Potential for a Research Career
- Sponsor's Biosketch (5 pages)
- Cosponsor's Biosketch (if required—5 pages)

Printed in the United States
By Bookmasters